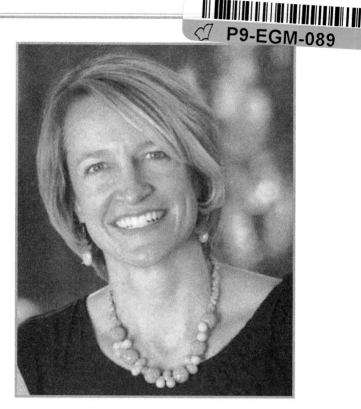

Red Sunshine

A STORY OF STRENGTH AND INSPIRATION
FROM A DOCTOR WHO SURVIVED
STAGE 3 BREAST CANCER

Kimberly Allison, M.D.

hatherleigh

Red Sunshine

Text Copyright © 2011 Kimberly Allison, M.D.

Hatherleigh Press is committed to preserving and protecting the natural resources of the Earth. Environmentally responsible and sustainable practices are embraced within the company's mission statement.

Hatherleigh Press is a member of the Publishers Earth Alliance, committed to preserving and protecting the natural resources of the planet while developing a sustainable business model for the book publishing industry.

This book was edited and designed in the village of Hobart, New York. Hobart is a community that has embraced books and publishing as a component of its livelihood. There are several unique bookstores in the village. For more information, please visit www.hobartbookvillage.com.

Library of Congress Cataloging-in-Publication Data
is available upon request.
ISBN 978-1-57826-407-0

Red Sunshine is available for bulk purchase, special promotions, and premiums. For information on reselling and special purchase opportunities, call 1-800-528-2550 and ask for the Special Sales Manager.

Cover and interior design by DCDesigns
Cover photo by Lisi Wolf, www.lisiwolf.com

10 9 8 7 6 5 4 3 2 1
Printed in the United States

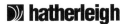

www.hatherleighpress.com

Red
Sunshine

A STORY OF STRENGTH AND INSPIRATION
FROM A DOCTOR WHO SURVIVED
STAGE 3 BREAST CANCER

Red Sunshine

"A moving memoir from a physician who became a patient with a very difficult diagnosis. This book offers an infusion of hope and inspiration for cancer survivors, regardless of their stage."

—*Julie Silver, M.D., Assistant Professor, Harvard Medical School and author of* What Helped Get Me Through: Cancer Survivors Share Wisdom and Hope

"Dr. Allison's perspective is both unique and familiar. As a breast cancer specialist, she knows all too well her prognosis and treatment plan as soon as she's diagnosed. She then embarks on an emotional journey through uncharted territory, warmly related in *Red Sunshine*. Her description is both heartfelt and down-to-earth. I'd recommend it to my patients as well as my colleagues."

—*Julie R. Gralow, M.D., Professor and Director, Breast Medical Oncology, Seattle Cancer Care Alliance and University of Washington Medical Center, Seattle, WA, Author of* Breast Fitness: An Optimal Exercise and Health Plan for Reducing Your Risk of Breast Cancer

"*Red Sunshine* is full of honesty, reflection, and information that people diagnosed with cancer, as well as those who support and treat them, will find so helpful. So many books sugar coat things but this memoir really gives a realistic picture of the experience and still manages to be funny, uplifting and a great read."

—*Kristine Calhoun, M.D., Breast Surgeon and Associate Professor, Seattle Cancer Care Alliance and University of Washington Medical Center, Seattle, WA*

"I could not put this book down. As a survivor myself, I was struck by the similarities in our experiences with cancer; the fear, the determination to be here for our children, the love and support from friends and family and our willingness to explore a variety of traditional and non-traditional ways to heal our bodies and our minds."

—*Julie Wheelan, Director, Center for Integrative Health & Wellness, Marin General Hospital, Marin County, CA*

"This is a captivating book. Once you start reading, you won't be able to put it down. You will feel the fear, pain and anger Kim faces, along with the strength, and sometimes even humor, she is able to summon in her journey as a cancer patient. I know all too well what Dr. Allison went through, having lived through breast cancer myself, and this book would have been a good friend to have on that journey."

—*D.O., survivor, professor, and mother*

"Who else has literally looked directly at her own cancer and said, 'I am going to absolutely crush you!' *Red Sunshine* is the girlfriend's guide to kicking cancer's ass."

—*S.D., physician and mother*

"From assigning her friends as various gurus to help her through, to performing backyard magic, and dreaming of 'Barbie Boobs'—this book had me hooked because of her hilarious and creative perspective."

—*S.K., survivor*

"Her voice is at once familiar. I felt like I had a new girlfriend that I wanted to call up and talk to about my diagnosis."

—*M.K., survivor*

"Reading your memoir was like being given an opportunity to peek into your soul—it means a great deal for someone like me who is at the brink of the treatment pathway with the great unknowns. I feel good for the first time after receiving my diagnosis."

—*A.S., physician and mother of twins, diagnosed at age 36*

"A must-read for anyone with cancer or who knows someone with that diagnosis. It is beautiful, poignant, humorous, and real."

—*A.M., supporter of a breast cancer survivor*

"When your doctor is advising you on a serious health issue it's so easy to think, 'Easy for you to say, buddy!' Well, the doctor is in the patient's shoes in *Red Sunshine* and that is what makes it such a great read. Dr. Allison is honest and clear-sighted, but this is no angsty cancer memoir. She is in a place of privilege when it comes to medical knowledge and connections, but has the good sense to know that all that knowledge and all those connections can't change her diagnosis. She also knows that it is up to her how she responds and she does so with grace, dignity, and wit. I recommend this for both doctors and patients."

—*Debra Jarvis, author of* It's Not About the Hair:
And Other Certainties of Life & Cancer

Contents

To all my co-survivors:
Keep living and learning

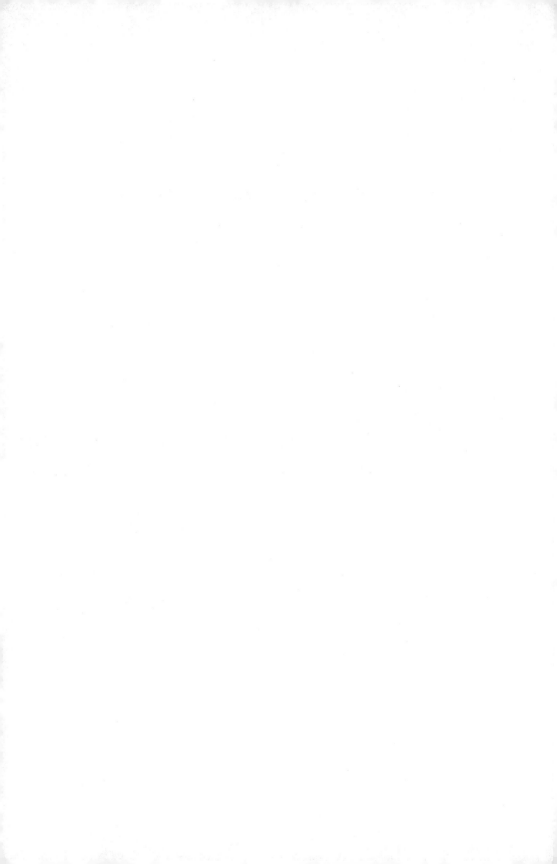

Foreword

"KIM HAS BREAST CANCER and wants you to be her surgeon." This was probably the last thing I expected to hear during the middle of an otherwise routine day in the operating room. My pager had gone off earlier during a procedure, and when the circulating nurse said it was a call from pathology, I thought it could wait. Usually, pathology pages me with results that I can respond to after a surgery is over. But when the nurse told me what the message was, I was shocked. Kim Allison, who only weeks ago had been appointed as our new Breast Pathology director when her prior mentor left, and who had a young daughter and infant son, had breast cancer and wanted me to be a member of her treatment team. I had treated other individuals I knew personally, including a number of nurses and the mother-in-law of one of my good friends, but Kim's diagnosis affected me on a more personal level. She was someone I saw multiple times a week, someone I relied on to do my job well, and she was close to my age. So many questions went through my mind—what if something went wrong with her surgery, what if she didn't respond well to treatment, would she be able to continue to work with the very disease that she was fighting? Mostly, though, I was worried that she would come to regret having treatment where she worked and would wish she had kept her personal and professional lives separate. We all gave her ample opportunities to seek care elsewhere, even providing the names of medical, surgical, and radiation oncologists for second opinions, but she declined. I was flattered when she chose me to be her surgeon, but also a little worried she would regret it at some point.

Fortunately, my misgivings proved to be wrong and I learned a lot from watching Kim navigate her course of treatment. Unlike most of my patients, I was exposed to so much more of Kim's journey than the initial consultation, the surgery, and the post-operative care. I saw her lose her hair, heard about the University of Washington men's crew team wearing pink shirts in her honor, laughed when she told me about Henry's reaction to her wigs, and saw how supportive her family was. Reading *Red Sunshine*, however, taught me so much more about her experience and opened my eyes to what my patients must experience when dealing with the whole process of a cancer diagnosis. Unlike most books about cancer, which read like "how-to" manuals of what to do, which questions to ask, how many opinions to obtain, and how to make treatment decisions, this account is much more personal and fills a needed void for those individuals unlikely to seek out a support group. I deal with breast cancer daily, but had never truly appreciated how much of what I say will be remembered by the patient. Kim taught me that encouraging statements are so much more than a cliché to a patient, something I will always remember in the future.

Red Sunshine is an intense, personal, and bluntly honest account of one woman's battle with breast cancer, written with an openness few would be willing to share with strangers, but I am so glad that she did. Although Kim's specific disease was breast cancer, the emotions, experiences, and situations that she recounts are applicable to anyone—male or female, young or old, patient or caregiver—beginning a journey with cancer. Kim told me she wanted to share her unique experience with others, specifically how she felt at certain times along the trail, so that others might not feel alone as they embark on their own path. Mission accomplished, Kim, mission accomplished.

—*Kristine Calhoun, M.D.,*
Breast Surgeon and Associate Professor, Seattle Cancer Care
Alliance and University of Washington Medical Center

Introduction

WHEN I WAS FIRST diagnosed with cancer, I had a burning
desire to know more. I surfed the Internet, cruised the bookstores, and made phone calls looking for answers to my questions.
As a pathologist who diagnoses and studies breast cancer, I already
knew a lot about what tests I would get, what sorts of treatments
were available, and what the survival statistics were. And there were
plenty of nice references available on cancer and advice books on
how to deal with it. But what I *really* wanted to know was what it
would be *like* to go through cancer treatment. How would it really
feel the first time I was hooked up to chemotherapy or lay still for
radiation? What was it like to be wheeled into the operating room,
and how much pain would I be in when I woke up? How would I
deal with continuing to raise my two young kids? How would I *not*
hit bottom and what would it be like when I inevitably did? Not just
would I survive, but *how* would I survive?

I wanted to hear from survivors. I wanted to know their stories
and feel their experiences and look for hidden clues to what my
future held. It was the story of a survivor, not all the medical statistics and research trials, which held the most value to me. Despite
the M.D. behind my name, this book is not meant to offer medical
advice or recommendations. It is only intended to share with you
what it was like for me to go through this experience. Everyone's
experience with cancer is completely unique and there is no right or

wrong way to go through it. But our stories connect us to a common core and can give us comfort that at least we are not alone in the experience.

Everyone has a story to tell.

This is mine.

KIMBERLY ALLISON, M.D.

Red
Sunshine

A STORY OF STRENGTH AND INSPIRATION
FROM A DOCTOR WHO SURVIVED
STAGE 3 BREAST CANCER

Bad Day at the Office

THE MORNING CHAOS IS in full swing. I am trying not to spill my latte as I unpeel my tearful seven-month-old from my arms and into the nanny's and usher my four-year-old to the car. Maddy is moving at her typical toddler pace, looking up at the sky and noticing the shape of the clouds, the squirrel in the tree, a broken toy next to our garbage. I am gently pushing her forward toward the already open car door.

"Let's not be late, honey," I say, trying not to sound too rushed. She has an uncanny ability to sense stress, which if detected, inevitably results in tears and tantrums that slow the whole ballgame down.

"Are we late, Mom?" she asks, testing the waters.

"Not yet, baby; let's just keep movin.'"

She gets buckled up. I realize I forgot my pager and rush back inside with the car running to get it.

"Have a good one, babe," Ryan, my husband, says as I whizz by him. He has been up since 4:00 AM at his new restaurant, getting things organized for the day and is back only to check e-mails and deliver me a coffee before he spends the rest of the day trying to make his struggling new business work. We hardly see each other since it opened. I never know if he will be home before dinner or to tuck the kids in at night. Neither of us are really sure how this all happened and how it was so awfully timed with Henry being born around the same time as the new business. I keep telling myself it will get better next month, but we are both clearly burning the candle at both ends.

I blow him a kiss on my way back out the door.

"I'll call you," I add, as I leave, and think about how he better be home for dinner tonight.

Maddy and I wave to Ryan as we pull out of the driveway and I head to preschool drop off. I watch as my daughter makes her way from my car-side good-bye hug to the preschool gate. I love watching this moment in-between safe havens—the thirty seconds when this tiny little person, toting a Scooby Doo lunch box, is truly independently navigating her world. She makes it to the gate and turns to wave.

I rush off down the road already thinking about my workday. Work has been crazy the last few weeks. Our primary breast cancer pathologist unexpectedly left and my chairman suddenly appointed me (with all of two years' experience) as the director of the breast pathology service. I really want to do a good job but at the same time feel nervously unprepared. I've really got to prove myself to the clinical team that I interact with in the next few months. I have to show them I can handle running the service and that they can trust my diagnoses without my previous mentor around to consult with.

When I get to the office, I find the resident on my service, and we settle down on opposite sides of my double-headed microscope to look at the cases for the day.

"This patient is a thirty-six year old with a breast mass and an abnormal lymph node on imaging," the resident tells me as I slip the glass biopsy slide onto the stage of my microscope.

It is not good news. Her biopsy has ugly sheets of cells traveling through her breast tissue in a disorganized way that is characteristic of malignancy.

"So what's your diagnosis?" I ask as I look at the pathology report the resident has written up.

"Invasive ductal carcinoma. Nottingham grade 3 because of poor tubule formation, high nuclear grade and high mitotic rate. We need to order the breast panel for the estrogen, progesterone, and HER2 stains, right?" she adds, referring to the additional studies we always perform on new diagnoses of breast cancer.

"Correct," I answer as I finalize the report and order the additional stains. I pause and think about that woman for a moment. Thirty-six years old and about to have her world turned completely upside down because of a breast cancer diagnosis. The radiologist who took the biopsy will receive my faxed report and deliver the news. I never even meet the patient. But I can't help but wonder about her. How will she take the news? How much will her life change because of what I just said in my report?

I do take pride in making the right diagnosis for her because I know that each woman's entire treatment plan will be tailored around the details that I report about their cancer. One woman's breast cancer may closely mimic normal breast tissue, forming beautifully structured glands, but only telling me that it is cancer because they are trickling through normal areas in subtly invasive ways. These cancers are bland and slow growing. Another woman's cancer can be so disorganized and confused that it is made up of nothing but ugly purple cells that grow in sheets like a big dark storm cloud. These are the aggressive "bad-ass" cancers. Both cancers can be lethal if untreated, but one might take ten to twenty years and the other less than a year. The treatments can be dramatically different too, with the slow-growing cancer responding well to hormonal therapy and the bad-ass one requiring several months of aggressive chemotherapy. Every woman's cancer is as unique as they are, and while I don't get to know the women, I get to know their cancers well enough that I can guide their surgeons and oncologists in their treatment decisions. Strange, I know. Who wants to know someone's cancer well?

But I love my job. I especially love my microscope. Looking through it is like looking through a keyhole to another universe, one where cells are suspended in time and stained beautiful purples and pinks. Some cancers are strangely beautiful, and I take pride in figuring out the details of their existence. My cases are nature's cellular hieroglyphics and I am their translator. And I know that nature is not perfect and can make mistakes.

I do think about the patients though, sometimes lingering on the details I learn about their personal history. *Just back from a trip to Disneyland with her family, and she finds out her cancer has recurred. Trying to get pregnant and finding a lump in her breast. Her husband just died and now she has cancer too.*

I especially think about the women similar to me in age, young mothers, some still even breast feeding, like I am. God, how awful would that be? Eyes closed, I swim to the mossy bottom of my mind and temporarily feel the slippery thoughts of these dark possibilities. What would she tell her children? Her husband? What would her treatment be like? Her future? Bumping up against these thoughts in the murky depths, they feel cold and implausible, but I play out the scenario just the same.

Diagnosing this young woman reminds me that I should go make an appointment with my doctor. I am slowing down breast feeding now that Henry is seven months old. Having to pump at work several times a day is getting old, and he likes the bottle any-way at this point. But now that I have slowed down breast feeding, I have noticed that there is a firmer area in the upper aspect of my left breast that stays up slightly higher than the right; it is a funny shelf-like area, not a lump. Ryan keeps reminding me to go get it checked. I know it is probably just nonproductive breast tissue—lazy breast buds. After all, most breast feeding lumps and bumps were nothing but plugged ducts or mastitis. And I am young and healthy with no family history of breast cancer at all. I am training for a half mara-thon and have never felt better, never better.

But I should call and make an appointment, just in case.

❖   ❖   ❖

TEN DAYS LATER I am walking my own breast biopsy down the hallway. A tiny, worm-shaped piece of me is floating in formalin in a little plastic jar with an orange top. I never thought I would see my own name on one of these labels, but there it is, "Kimberly Allison, 33 y F" with my patient identification number listed afterwards. This feels so surreal but also a little like a strange lab experiment. I'm just trying this out for fun, I tell myself.

My doctor didn't like what she saw when I came in to see her a few days ago. She especially didn't like that the area was hard and not easily movable. I reminded her that sometimes *both* of my breasts were hard and immovable—I was breast feeding after all (the one time in my life when I was actually well endowed!). She ordered me a mammogram, which was a complete storm of white since I was still lactating—no help at all. So I was sent for an ultrasound, and there they saw a pretty large mass lurking. The radiologist was a colleague, and we chatted about working on a research project together while he searched around with his ultrasound wand. Another, more senior, radiologist came in as well. She didn't sound too worried, reminding me that most breast changes during lactation are benign but told me we could biopsy.

"Of course I want a biopsy! I want to look at it!" I quip. And I really did want to see what it would be like to look at my own *benign* breast tissue under the microscope. This couldn't possibly be cancer anyway. That would just be too ironic—a breast pathologist who diagnoses breast cancer all day gets cancer herself.

Now here I am holding that very biopsy in my hands. I am fairly confident it is nothing to worry about. I hand the jar off to our physician's assistant and tell him this is my own biopsy and I want it to bypass the resident training with us this time for privacy but that I am really not worried. So don't worry.

I let one of my colleagues know she will be seeing my biopsy this morning and to let me know when she is ready for me to look at it. I tell her how *not* worried I am. I go back to my office and sit at my microscope. *This was all just an experiment about what it would be like to be on the other side of the microscope, right?* I have diagnosed breast cancer in women in their thirties many times, but that was not my story—no sir, not me.

The morning was passing away rapidly. The slides from my biopsy must be out by now. I peek out of my office and see my colleague's door is closed. *Hmm . . . Should I be worried about this delay? No, she is just busy.* Finally, I hear a knock on my door, and in peeks both the colleague who was reading out my biopsy and another friend and colleague, Rochelle, both with serious looks on their faces.

I smile and say "About time!"

Then I realize Rochelle is usually working at another hospital today. "What are you doing here?" I ask innocently, and as soon as the words leave my mouth, I realize she has come to help deliver bad news.

"Holy crap. No. It's cancer isn't it?" I manage quickly.

They nod. They start to cry.

"What?" I don't understand. Why are these women crying in my office? These women that trained me and I work with professionally. Why am I not crying? I am suddenly starving for information.

"Is it a grade 3? Crap, if this is cancer then it is huge! What stage am I?"

And in a matter of only a few seconds I am realizing what I will go through in the next year.

"This is bad. I'm going to need chemotherapy. I'm going to have a mastectomy. And I'm going to go through menopause." I blurt out numbly.

I try to be funny or find something good about the situation, but there really is nothing I can spin off this one. I feel bad for my colleagues. They should not have to tell me I have cancer. They cry harder than me at first.

Then I think of my children. They are so young, four years old and seven months—too young to see their mother go through this, too young to lose me. I watch my dreams of a third child fizzle and turn to ash. And my poor husband, who lost both his only brother and his father too young, he can't possibly lose a wife as well.

I finally start to cry. And my shoulders are shaking with the strength of the downpour. I feel like Alice in Wonderland with everything in the room suddenly upside down, too big or too small. The world just doesn't make sense anymore. I need to wake up and realize I am in a dream world of an alternate reality. But there is no waking from this strange dream and I keep crying and crying.

"OK. What do I do?" I ask out loud when I finally come up for air.

"You call Ryan and have him come pick you up. Do you want me to call one of the breast oncologists and a surgeon for you to talk to?" said Rochelle.

Fuck. I need an oncologist and a surgeon. I want them here right now telling me it is going to be all right, we will remove your breast today and you will continue on with life. I know our hospital's breast surgeons and oncologists well since I present the pathology of all the breast cancer patients at our tumor boards. They are the ones I am supposed to be impressing with my ability to diagnose their patients well, so they know how to best treat them. We are about to get to know each other on a whole other level.

Ryan comes to pick me up. I call him and simply say, "I have a really bad breast cancer and I need you to come pick me up." No sugar-coating this one. He was there in a flash, shell-shocked and supportive. I could have done this lighter. Poor guy has had too many bad emergency phone calls in his life already. His younger brother died in a car crash at nineteen, and his father died of a sudden heart attack at age fifty. But I have no way to break this lightly. I know it is serious, and I want him to know too.

We just drive around and try to digest things. We talk about our plan of action. We make phone calls and appointments. He is confused and scared and so am I. But I am starting to find silver linings to share with him.

"At least it is something potentially curable."

"At least we caught it now."

"At least I know all the people involved in my care."

And importantly, at least we have each other. I have been so lucky in so many ways. I love my husband, kids, and job.

Now I am holding my breath and waiting for things to fall apart.

Slow Car Crash

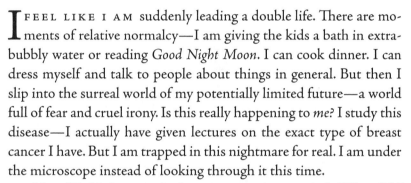

I FEEL LIKE I AM suddenly leading a double life. There are moments of relative normalcy—I am giving the kids a bath in extra-bubbly water or reading *Good Night Moon*. I can cook dinner. I can dress myself and talk to people about things in general. But then I slip into the surreal world of my potentially limited future—a world full of fear and cruel irony. Is this really happening to *me*? I study this disease—I actually have given lectures on the exact type of breast cancer I have. But I am trapped in this nightmare for real. I am under the microscope instead of looking through it this time.

How did this happen? And ever present in my mind: *What did I do wrong?* My mind keeps searching desperately for an explanation.

The fairly logical explanations go first:
> *It must be some toxin in the water.*
> *It must be the stress.*
> *It must be the lack of sunshine in the Northwest.*
> *Is it my genes?*
> *Was it the pregnancy?*

And the illogical ones:
> *Is this some kind of cruel payback?*
> *A curse?*
> *Some Jedi mind trick?*

It is the end of March, and the usually drab Seattle weather has taken a turn as bizarre as my life feels. Hail suddenly interrupts sunny skies, and rainbows intermix with snow showers. Nothing feels real except my fear. And it is my fear that keeps me circling in another orbit. It grips me constantly and with a strength that makes me physically shake on a regular basis.

I think I can survive the initial treatment plan. It is my *long-term* survival I am now fearing the most. What is my prognosis exactly?

I have a high grade (bad-ass), hormone-receptor negative (bad-ass), lymph node positive (bad-ass), 7 cm (big and bad-ass), pregnancy-associated (also bad), invasive ductal carcinoma that overexpresses a protein called Her2 (take a guess—also bad-ass). I know all too well that none of this is considered favorable. I try to tell myself it could be worse (although it is really hard to buy it at this point). My cancer is still considered potentially curable because there is no definite sign that it has spread to distant organs. But really it is considered locally advanced and aggressive—not much positive about it, and I know it. So I am scared to death to look up the actual statistics on my prognosis, but I know I want the information.

Ahhh . . . the dangerous abyss of the Internet—so much information with so little filter. It seems custom designed just to freak out a newly diagnosed cancer patient. At least I can read through studies with some degree of medical acumen, but even so I get pretty terrified looking at the ones on breast cancers associated with a recent pregnancy. I keep trying to remind myself that most of these studies are old and there are new treatments available now. I *know* all this, but I still keep desperately searching for the study or Web site that will tell me all will be well. I spend fruitless hours pouring over the data, trying to find the answer I want: Not just how many survive, but will *I* survive. Of course, that answer is not available by any current modern technology.

I go to the online database I know will give me one of the most medically reliable answers and punch in my data. So many unfavorable features, plus my young age, I am bracing myself for the statisti-

cal fortune-teller to predict my grim future, and it does. About a 40
percent ten-year survival rate is what it quotes me. I sit very still and
feel my heart pounding in my chest with an irregular throbbing. So
basically, it is worse than a flip of the coin—not great odds. I try to
tell myself that at least they are close to 50 percent. And these are just
statistics. What does it matter if you have a 95 percent mortality rate
if you are in that lucky 5 percent that survives? Still, I am feeling very
sober and am having trouble not shaking visibly.

"You OK?" Ryan asks concerned, as he sees me wide-eyed staring at the computer screen of my laptop. But I can't really answer at
that moment. I am retreating to a dead-woman-walking state where
all I can think of is what life will be like for everyone without me.

Ryan keeps watching the TV.

I am slowly dying on the couch and the world is going on without me already.

That night I dream that I am in a slow-motion car crash. The
initial impact sets me in a rapid tailspin, but then the liquid space of
the dream thickens and I watch helplessly as little shards of the car
are slowly torn away from me. I wake up unable to shake the feeling
that my future is also slowly being torn from me, one painful injury
at a time.

When I am not numbly floating in this purgatory, in-between
the living and the dead, then I am in panic mode. I want to get this
taken care of right away. I think of every little malignant cell continuing to divide in my body like a ticking time bomb. Maybe one has
finally decided to set up shop somewhere awful like my lungs, liver,
or bones. I can picture them spinning through my blood stream,
looking for a new home. I know I have to wait to see my doctors
until most of the information they need to make a plan is gathered,
but it is so hard to wait in this purgatory. And I know that the cancer
has probably been there for months at least and a few more days
would not likely make any difference in my survival. But that doesn't
help the anxiety. I want someone to hold my hand and tell me the
plan *today*. I get another biopsy of an abnormal appearing lymph

node and wait for the results nervously, just like my patients do. The cancer is in the lymph node too. Tick. Tick.

At last I meet with my team. I love my team. Since I have worked with them for the past few years, I know my surgeon, oncologist, and radiation oncologist fairly well already. I wanted to stay where I worked because I considered it one of the best places in the United States to be treated and I had the benefit of knowing everyone involved. This wasn't like when I had my babies, when I didn't really want to have the doctor who saw me in the cafeteria having to be checking on my "girl parts" as they contorted to perform the amazingly animal act of childbirth. This time my privacy is not the issue, my survival is.

So today the whole team is meeting with Ryan and me all at once, to establish our plan of attack. I open the door to a conference room and there they are, not waiting to hear my opinion on a biopsy, but waiting to tell *me* what *my* treatment plan will be. I am still not used to being on the other side of the table, but I try to look confident and upbeat. They run through their treatment scenarios and I ask questions.

I feel comfortable talking about all the medical options because I feel so familiar with them. I have to say, you *do* think about what you would do if you were the patient when you are diagnosing cancer on a daily basis, so I had some opinions already about surgery, etc. Ryan sits quietly and waits for someone to translate the medical mumbo jumbo we are throwing around. We come to a treatment plan. Because my cancer is so large and appears to have already spread to at least one lymph, we will treat it with six months of chemotherapy first (neoadjuvantly), both in the hopes of killing off up-front any microscopic cancer that has secretly spread to other sites and to see how my cancer responds to therapy. So my initial instinct to "lop it off" will have to wait until the fall. My chemo weapons of choice will be weekly Adriamycin (a "big gun" chemotherapy agent with lots of toxicities) and daily oral Cytoxan for three months and then weekly

Taxol for the second three months along with an antibody therapy called Herceptin, which I will receive for a year.

In the fall I will need a modified radical mastectomy, a surgery removing both my breast and the lymph nodes under my armpit. I can't have a lumpectomy, where only a part of the breast is removed, because my breasts are small and the cancer is large. Actually, I am leaning towards having both breasts removed (despite my surgeon telling me it is not medically necessary to do so). First of all, who wants one perky reconstructed boob and one tiny droopy one? I consider them a set. And my post-breast-feeding size is not exactly something I would show off. They have basically become tiny deflated bags of skin—not a sexy visual, I know. There are plenty of surgical tricks to provide symmetry these days, which I am also willing to consider, but I have no problem with a complete replacement set. Second, I am young and with a breast cancer diagnosis so early in my hopefully long life, I am at a higher lifetime risk of a second breast cancer. So either I sign up for a lifetime of close screening, which can usually detect even very small cancers, or I try to surgically minimize the risk up-front. According to the literature out there, since I have a poor-prognosis cancer my overall survival from this cancer will not be altered by having the opposite breast removed. This is a personal choice and I know it would be different for every woman. I will also be tested for mutations in the breast cancer genes *BRCA1* and *BRCA2*, the results of which will play a role in my decision since, if I test positive, the lifetime risk of cancer in the opposite breast increases dramatically.

To top off my treatment battle plan, I will get post-mastectomy radiation. This is mainly because of a study that showed that women with locally advanced breast cancer like mine reduced their recurrence rates with radiation. I don't think there is a therapeutic modality that I will *not* be getting! I will get "the works." I am happy to be throwing everything but the kitchen sink at this cancer, as long as we think it will work. *It has to work, right?*

My surgeon, a young dynamo of a woman, is comforting me with her optimism.

"This is the kind of breast cancer that responds really well to treatment, Kim." I think that one over. *She is right; the aggressive cancers can respond really well and even disappear completely if you are lucky.*

"We're talking about seeing your grandkids here." She says.

I immediately tear up at the thought. Really?

My oncologist is quiet, making no promises.

I know there are no guarantees, but I had never doubted my ability to live to see my grandchildren before. Now I am thinking seeing the grandkids would be an amazing privilege.

The Club

A FEW DAYS AFTER I am diagnosed I find myself in the elevator at the cancer center with the chairman of my department. He is being treated here as a patient as well, but he has no idea that I am not here for work. He has endured two cancer diagnoses and a stem cell transplant—tough stuff. Only weeks ago, after our main breast pathologist left unexpectedly, he gave me the title of director of breast pathology, and I want him to know things are going well in my hands. But he also needs to know my diagnosis.

The elevator is crowded. I say hello and he nods. Out of nowhere I burst out with "I'm here as a patient." He looks confused and says yes, he is here as a patient. "No, I am here as a patient too."

"What diagnosis?" he asks with some disbelief.

"Breast cancer," I say and am embarrassed that I start to cry. I have not said this too many times out loud yet, and it still makes me emotional.

The elevator is painfully silent and when the doors open we step aside.

"In situ carcinoma?" he asks hopefully. In situ carcinoma is the kind that has not yet invaded so cannot spread.

"No, grade 3 invasive carcinoma." I sigh.

He pats me on the back and says, "Well, welcome to the club."

Just what I wanted, to be a member of an exclusive club with the chairman of my department. I picture us drinking antioxidant smoothies over chemotherapy, laughing with our knit caps on our bald heads and IV poles hanging toxic chemicals beside us. What a strange irony. I am probably one of the youngest members of the department and he is one of the oldest. Yet here we are together discussing our cancer club.

I look around at the patients in the lobby. Everyone looks so dull and ashen. Only a rare face looks as young as I am in this sea of moans and groans. *Am I going to become one of them?—a faded, depressing version of myself?* Suddenly I want to talk to other young women with breast cancer. I have to find them and have them tell me it will be OK.

And somehow, they find me. An ex-girlfriend of a friend who was also thirty-three when she was diagnosed, only months before she was to be married. She had a bilateral mastectomy instead of her wedding day. Another woman my mother works with who was diagnosed the day she gave birth to her second child with a breast cancer that had already spread to other organs. A friend's sister-in-law was diagnosed while nursing her third child. Another friend's relative was diagnosed two years after having twins. I am starving for their stories, their tips and experiences, and they feed me every morsel I ask for. None of them are in the same city, so I hold their hands from a distance and they comfort me over the phone and e-mail. I am so thankful for them. They tell me I can do this—that it is not an insurmountable task. They tell me the chemotherapy is not all that bad, that I can have a wig made of my own hair or wear stylish scarves, that I don't have to have a "good attitude," that I don't have to never hug my kids again without worrying about what germs they will be giving me while I'm on chemotherapy, and that the treatments will end and life will go on.

I know I can start this journey now. I still find myself shaking unexpectedly with the nervous anticipation of the unknown. But I am actually excited now to start chemotherapy. I want to go to battle and start fighting the storm cloud that was secretly brewing in my body—blast it into pieces. I decide chemo is going to be my friend, my weapon of choice. It feels empowering. That's what this club is, not a club of the sick and weak but of bare-headed warriors, and it is an honor to join their ranks.

Did Chocolate Do This?

I AM SCHEDULED FOR MY first dose of chemotherapy this Wednesday and am happy with my medical treatment plan and team, but I feel like I need a personal action plan as well. I decide I need a team of gurus to help me through this. Other "pink" ladies have warned me: If you don't assign people jobs, they will still want to help out and you might get help in ways that you really didn't want. Plus, it makes the people who care about you feel good to be part of your healing team. We are not talking about major jobs here. I figure even just a guru title is enough to make them feel included.

My girlfriend from high school, Sheila, will be my music guru, tasked with making the soundtrack to get me through chemotherapy sessions. She is a master of tunes, and back in high school her mix tapes were always crystallizing our latest moods in music. Jessica, a good friend here in Seattle who is a Charlize Theron look-a-like and is always dressed in perfect style, will be my cancer-fashion guru. She is already collecting recommendations on where to get a wig made of my own hair and compiling a chemo kit stocked with false eyelashes and the best eyebrow pencil available. Naomi is my "check on my parents" guru, since she lives near them in California (I know she will do much more than that because, for a friend in need, she has no limits). Joanna, who lives in London, is my international guru. Neither of us knows exactly what that means, but it feels really good to have someone on another continent cheering for me anyway. I don't have a fitness guru, but I need one because I know I want to stay in decent physical condition, so I sign up for yoga classes and weight-circuit training (not all gurus are free).

And I assign my close friend Claudia to be my nutrition guru. Claudia is a preppy Seattle environmental lawyer (originally from St. Louis). A math and philosophy major in college and voracious reader, she is totally game for additional research. Our families are really closely intertwined because our husbands and kids are all good friends. Some weekends we have what we jokingly call "commune" weekends when we basically spend the whole weekend at each other's houses alternating who goes and runs errands while the kids are playing together. Although when it comes to cooking meals, our husbands are the kings of the kitchen (lucky us!), we are the ones who make sure we don't eat crab and steak with blue cheese every night and that the kids are eating healthy, well-balanced meals. She is already well-versed on the so-called "Super Foods," has some crazy green drink for breakfast in the morning, and is excited to be assigned as nutrition guru. What anti-cancer or anti-chemo-side-effects diet should I be on?

She is quickly at my house armed with books on nutrition and cancer hot off the shelves. We browse through the pages quickly looking for the take-home messages. Several of them are full of messages about sugar feeding cancer and how to make our bodies more alkaline because cancer likes an acidic environment. Pretty much they recommend eating nothing but veggies pulled straight from the earth and blended in a juicer.

No problem. Next stop: my local natural foods store.

We browse the aisles picking up anything that seems to meet our qualifications, buying ingredients for green drinks and protein shakes. But we really have no clue what we are doing. I look at my grocery cart filled with kale as we are checking out with a lump in my throat and think *I have no idea how to cook kale. What am I going to do with all this stuff?* Claudia and I look at each other over our antioxidant-rich feast and break down in laughter.

Nevertheless, I take it all home and blend things and try a sip of a frothy veggie puree that tastes like sea foam. I enviously watch my husband eat desert and drink wine that night. *This just doesn't seem fair, I have a potentially limited future and I don't even get to enjoy treats anymore?* The lump in my throat returns. Why am I not being more critical and scientific about this dietary change? Somehow, when you have cancer you are so worried that you have done something wrong or are doing something wrong, you are willing to believe in anything.

I soon realize that I haven't really thought this through. In fact, I really don't understand the argument that sugar preferentially feeds cancer. Glucose feeds all our cells and is what most fuel we eat is broken down into. Specialized scans to look for metabolic activity done with radio-labeled glucose do show increased uptake in the areas of cancer, but that is because cancers are such hungry monsters. If you radio-labeled any starchy vegetable, they would do the same thing, since they are broken down into glucose eventually. Take away all your blood sugar and your brain will starve since it runs purely on glucose (hence the diabetic coma when a diabetic takes too much insulin and their blood sugar drops.) Too much refined sugar is of course not ideal either because the fuel is used too fast or not stored well, but cancer patients need to have calories to keep their bodies running because cancers are like little parasites, taking what they want for fuel and dividing like mad. They don't care if you are trying to starve them of sugar, they will take what they need so the rest of you starves (which is why cancers often make you lose weight). And they don't "like" an acidic environment; instead, they actually *make* one because they often resort to anaerobic metabolism to survive when there is no oxygen around them to fuel them. So, do I *really* have to totally give up chocolate? Come on now!

I decide that moderation is key. I do believe nutrition is important and eating sugar and fat all day is not the key to health. Eating healthy will keep my whole body and immune system strong. But I always considered myself a healthy eater. I grew up in California after all, so I am well-trained in eating organic veggies and low-fat foods. I need to give myself a break here. I did not get cancer because I ate unhealthy foods. I think in my case it is just really bad luck. My immune surveillance was down because of pregnancy, and there was a bad cell division mistake, and my body didn't recognize it in time to fix it before it grew beyond normal controls. So instead of feeling incredibly guilty about anything I eat that may not be on the "A" list of vegan purists, I decide to stop beating myself up. A piece of chocolate is not suicide. I do give up my nightly ice cream ritual and try to crank up the volume on my fresh veggies and fruits. I even start juicing. But come on, a girl can only do so much.

Facing the Red Sunshine

M Y FIRST WEEK POST-DIAGNOSIS has been filled with extra tests and appointments. I learn that getting a CT scan with contrast makes you feel like you have to pee really bad for a few minutes as the contrast filters into your pelvic area. I get some of my blood radioactively labeled to get a heart scan called a MUGA, to check my baseline cardiac status since the type of chemotherapy I will be on actually can kill off heart muscle. And I will get a bone scan to make sure the cancer has not already spread to my bones.

Since the radiologist is in the room looking at my images, I ask him if he sees anything worrisome in the spooky-looking, shadowy skeleton on the screen. He asks if I am a runner because he sees increased signal in a part of my pelvis that runners often get, but he doesn't see anything indicative of bone metastases—finally some good news.

The other thing I do in the week since my diagnosis is stop breastfeeding . . . cold turkey. Man, I do *not* recommend this! I was planning on tapering off slowly over the next few months since Henry is now eight months old, but to just stop abruptly is like trying to stop going to the bathroom for a few days. I get so swollen and sore I have to walk around with ice packs in my bra and dose myself with Tylenol. I even give in and pump a few times just for some relief.

Henry is relatively fine with the change. He was already taking bottles while I was at work, and he adjusts to formula mixed with previously frozen breast milk just fine. I think about how I was feeding him all that time from a cancerous breast. Were there cancer cells floating around in the milk? I shudder not wanting to think about it but am relieved that there has never been a case of passing cancer on to a baby through breast feeding. Funny how pregnancy books are full of all sorts of foods to avoid when pregnant and breast feeding, but feeding a baby from a cancerous breast is harmless.

My first day of chemotherapy approaches. I will be getting Adriamycin (doxorubicin)—otherwise known as the "Red Devil" because of its bright red color and devilish side effects—intravenously. Adriamycin is a "heavy hitter" that can cause severe nausea, constipation, mouth sores, and serious drops in your white blood cells. Because it can be so immunosuppressive, I will be giving myself shots in the abdomen six nights a week with G-CSF, a growth factor that stimulates the bone marrow to make more white cells called neutrophils. The other drug I will take, Cytoxan (cyclophosphamide), is in pill form. I already have a jar full of round light blue pills that I will take every day for the next three months. My nurse warns me to wash my hands after handling the pills since, "they are chemotherapy after all." *Great, what will they be doing to my GI tract?!*

I decide to do some background reading on these two drugs in terms of their history. Where did these drugs come from? Cytoxan is basically a derivative of mustard gas. It is given as a pro-drug, which means it is only toxic once your body converts it into its active form—nasty stuff. But I am intrigued to learn that the Red Devil, Adriamycin, was developed from a red bacteria found in the soil next to a castle built in the Middle Ages in Spain. In the 1950s there was a commission to find more soil-based microbes with potential therapeutic benefit and this little red warrior was just lying around waiting to be discovered. It proved to have anti-cancer activity in vitro by interfering with cell division. Eventually, the key product of the bacteria was harnessed in the laboratory to churn out more massive amounts.

I find this story slightly romantic. The natural beginnings of this toxin strangely comfort me a bit . . . I guess. I will be getting a little taste of the Middle Ages. Hopefully, it won't be as bad as the Black Plague. It is a powerful drug that is not targeted in any way to the cancer, so my whole body will suffer along with the cancer. But I know it is my best shot at beating this thing, so I decide that I will not think of it as the enemy, but as my "Red Sunshine" helping to bring light to all the dark places in my body that the cancer cells could hide.

The drug I will be receiving for the second three months of my chemotherapy is called Taxol (paclitaxel). This drug also has natural beginnings. It is derived from the bark of the Pacific Yew tree, found only in old growth forests of the Pacific Northwest (my neck of the woods!). A 1960s initiative by the United States National Cancer Institute to discover plant-based chemotherapies, found that this tree's bark had anti-cancer properties. After the compound responsible for the anti-cancer properties was isolated, it was called Taxol, after the botanical name for the yew tree, *Taxus*.

Taxol's success in initial animal and human cancer trials in the 1980s actually led to quite an ethical and political controversy since the demand for Taxol threatened to both damage the fragile old growth forest ecosystem and lead to the extinction of the now-valuable tree. The problem was that a large quantity of the yew tree bark contained only a small amount of the active compound. Once it was figured out how to recreate the product in the lab from large cell culture systems, the drug could be produced in massive enough quantities to bring it efficiently to the market without threatening the environment. It wasn't until the 1990s that it was approved by the FDA to treat ovarian and breast cancers, over thirty years after it was first collected from the depths of that Pacific Northwest forest. Ironically, the same tree that Native Americans used to make harpoons and canoe paddles also holds a key ingredient to treating human cancers.

OK, enough medical history.

The big day approaches. I am strangely excited to get the show started. I really don't like knowing that I have a cancer thriving inside me and I'm not doing anything about it. So I am ready to dive in head first. But it also terrifies me. My only experience in medical school was on the inpatient oncology wards where only patients who had serious complications were. I had never seen oncology patients in the outpatient setting, much less seen an infusion center so I have no idea what to expect.

Will I be spending my days incapacitated in the bathroom? Will I be able to function as a mother? Keep working? What if I get a cold or the flu? With little ones at home, it almost seems unavoidable. Will I have to be living in a sterile bubble where my runny-nosed kids can't get near me? This is the side effect I am most worried about. Not losing my hair or my taste buds. But getting sick and losing the ability to snuggle with my kids. *That* would be cruel but feels almost inevitable at this point.

My nurse tries to reassure me and tells me, "If you get sick you will still have an immune system, and it will fight it. We only really worry when you have a fever because your bacteria-fighting neutrophils are hit the hardest."

OK, I guess I am not having a bone marrow transplant. My immune system will not be taken down to zero. I will not be living in a bubble unless things get really bad.

"We encourage you to get exercise during treatment as well. Studies have shown women have fewer side effects and less fatigue when they stay active," my nurse continues.

I make a mental pledge to stay active and actually go to those yoga classes and circuit-training sessions I signed up for. *What else should I be doing? What should I not be doing?* There are too many unanswered questions at this point. I just want to start getting this over with.

Ryan and I head up to the fifth floor where infusion takes place. All my time working here and I have never had a reason to go to this floor before. We hand my little green patient identification card to the woman smiling at the front desk and are told to take a seat. The waiting room area is beautiful, with floor-to-ceiling windows facing sunny skies over Lake Union. But the "customers" here are sullen and grim. Sunken faces hang under knit caps. One very thin young man is in a wheelchair. I still stand out in this crowd with my full head of hair and nervous energy. A woman with a pretty scarf on her head smiles at me and nods. Does she know it's my first time?

They call my name and give me a room number to head to. I try to walk with confidence past the automatic double-doors into "The Land of Infusion," wishing instead I was headed to the magical kingdom of Narnia. I think I would rather face the Snow Queen than the Red Devil. Ryan hates hospitals because they remind him of when his brother died so he is probably not doing much better.

I find our room number. A nice white hospital bed awaits me in a clean room with a window. The doors are sliding glass with additional curtains for privacy. Some of the rooms just have curtains without the glass doors. Do they want me in sound isolation in case I start screaming my first time?

A nurse offers me a warmed blanket. This seems quite luxurious and slows the nervous tremor I am suffering from. I try to tell myself I am here for a spa treatment. They take my vitals and my nurse introduces herself. We do some small talk as she checks out my IV and prepares paperwork. She starts dosing me with Aloxi, an IV anti-nausea pre-medication, and gives me two small steroid pills to swallow.

A pretty blonde woman with a coffee cup in hand knocks on the door. *Who is this?* She does not look like one of the nurses. Instead of scrubs she is wearing a hot little outfit with red boots, a colorful necklace, and matching earrings.

"Hi, I'm one of the hospital chaplains, Deborah Jarvis. Mind if I chat with you?" She smiles a big friendly smile.

I immediately stiffen. I was raised in the 1970s by two ex-Catholics who never pushed a specific traditional religion on me, thinking I could choose my own when I grew up if I wanted. But without a religious upbringing, I actually never developed an interest in joining a church or temple. In fact, it made me nervous to be there because I knew I wasn't officially "part of the club." So what are the motives of this hospital chaplain? I eye her suspiciously. *Is she going to try to convert me right here while I am trapped, hooked to an IV pole?*

But she just makes me comfortable with small talk and gives me light-hearted support. She is a recent breast cancer survivor too. We talk about the strangeness of being a patient when you are so used to being on the other side of things at work. I like her and her positive energy. She makes me feel OK about being here and she's not a downer. She does carefully bridge the topic of going to church and how supported it made her feel. But she must sense my tension with the topic and it is quickly dropped.

We are chatting so much that I hardly notice when my nurse tells me it is time to start my infusion. She is all gowned up in gloves and a blue full-body protective cover. She is holding a syringe filled with a fluid that looks exactly like cherry Kool-Aid.

"Why the gown?" I ask.

"Well, supposedly if we get any of the Adria on us, it can cause severe skin burns. So it's just a precaution," she answers cautiously.

Sweet. That's comforting. What will it do to my veins?

She pulls up a stool and hooks up the syringe to my IV. Very slowly she puts pressure on the end of the syringe so that a thin ribbon of red begins to travel down the tubing toward the IV in my hand. I am waiting for a burn or a wave of nausea. But I feel nothing. It is actually quite mesmerizing to watch the thin red stream flowing down the tubing. My fabulous chaplain keeps Ryan and me chatting, and before twenty minutes are up, the syringe is empty.

"That's it?" I ask in shock. I am feeling exactly the same as before the infusion, only a little less nervous. *I can do this.*

"That's it. The steroids we gave you will make you feel pretty good until about twenty-four hours from now. You will probably feel a let-down tomorrow afternoon. So be ready to be able to lay low at that time until you see how it affects you."

Ryan and I look at each other and smile. That was too easy. Some of my fellow survivors had warned me about how bad the first round can be before they have figured out how to dose side-effect medication for you. Whatever they gave me already seems to be working . . . at least so far.

I stop by the bathroom on the way out. With all the extra IV fluids they have given me, my bladder is really full. I have been forewarned that my urine would likely be a red-orange color after infusion and am curious if it can happen right away or if it takes a while to run through my kidneys. Sure enough the toilet water has turned the colors of a good sunset from my Red Sunshine. I smile, impressed. It is already in my system working away at the cancer.

Ryan and I go out for a nice lunch, and I feel fine. I joke about it being my last meal with taste buds intact. I am imagining the red juice running through me, finding my cancer and making those rapidly dividing cells freeze in their tracks. I think I can feel a burn in my left breast. *It is working. It is working.*

Then we go to Costco to get some errands done.

Life goes on.

The Day After

THAT EVENING I AM jazzed. The steroids make me want to organize, fix, and rearrange things. I get tasks done around the house. I make fancy little snacks for the kids. I rearrange the toy bins. I reorganize the pantry. My face is flushed like I have been running on a hot summer day. I am super-productive mom! I also begin the constant cancer-probing that I will continue for the next six months before surgery, always testing to see if things have changed. Is the cancer softer? Is the chemo working?

How about now?

Now?

Eventually, I calm myself enough to go to sleep that night.

The next day I wake up still intact and don't feel too worse for the wear physically. I drive Maddy to preschool and stand in the rain crying for twenty minutes telling another mom about what is going on. Maddy does not know yet, and I am waiting for the right time to tell her. They tell me I have at least two weeks before my hair falls out so I have a little time to plan it.

How do you explain cancer to a four-year-old? It all just seems a bit advanced for a four-year-old mind and way too heavy for my sensitive little creature. She feels empathy for an unintentionally squished ant on the sidewalk. She cried in mourning when she heard about her favorite bakery closing, asking dramatically, "But where did it *go*?" How is she going to deal with her mother having a life-threatening illness and losing all her hair? We will clearly have to handle this one lightly, but I am not up to it today. I want to see how things go with the first few weeks of chemotherapy. If it is not too bad, I won't have to explain it like I am going to be deathly ill for six months and scare the bejesus out of her.

The rest of the morning I hang out with my little guy, funny, handsome Henry. He is already a jokester at eight months. Not nearly as sensitive as his sister was at his age (she would cry when an airplane made noise as it passed overhead, while he screams with excitement). He amazes me with his constant happiness and ability to turn anything, even the toast I give him for breakfast, into a car that moves to his little machine-mouth noises.

And I don't mean to brag, but *man* is he handsome! He already knows his giant blue eyes work wonders on me. I even find myself blushing sometimes or fixing my hair when he smiles up at me. I literally want to eat that vanilla baby right up and am constantly rubbing cheeks and kissing his soft white-gold head. His big sister amazingly feels the same way. Their four-year-age gap and her empathetic nature have made for much less jealousy than I remember feeling when my little brother was born. The love she feels for him is so passionate that she sometimes has trouble controlling it, and I can see her wanting to hug him a little too tight or rubbing his cheek softly but with her teeth clenched. Once she even took a tender bite of his ear and when she saw his reaction to the pain she caused, she ran screaming and crying to her room in self-punishment (and Mom's angry scolding). But honestly, I don't blame her for wanting to try to consume him. He does look absolutely delicious.

The day goes on and I keep waiting for the horrible nausea to send me reeling. Or my taste buds to suddenly dry up like evaporating dew. When will I be bedridden? It is not until late that afternoon that I finally feel some effects.

We are all gathered in the living room and I am suddenly aware of the steroids wearing off. A deep wave of fatigue comes over me, and I am rather abruptly sinking deep into a snowbank of sleepiness. My eyelids are extraordinarily heavy and it takes great effort to just keep them at half-mast. It feels like someone has brought kryptonite into the room and with each minute I am losing my powers. I try to fight it. I remember my nurse telling me it is good to stay active to avoid side effects. I get up off the couch and try walking around. I go outside for some fresh air. But *man* is my wagon draggin'.

"Why don't you go lie down and take a nap, Kim?" Ryan tells me, as he witnesses my struggle.

No, no. I must stay awake.

For some reason, I feel like if I can fight off this drowsy undertow I will survive. I want to stay in the game and not check out. I know I should give myself a break, but I want to be *alive*, not asleep like a dead girl. I remember when I first saw my newborn daughter as the doctor lifted her up for me to see. She was screaming and wiggling and red. I was shocked to see such expressive vitality after knowing her as a peaceful tumbler in my belly, so the first words that came out of my mouth were, "It's *alive!*" I need now to wiggle and scream with vitality. To move around means to know I am still here and still breathing.

And slowly, the wave passes through me. As I move around I reawaken and am able to continue on with the rest of my menial day. But I feel like I conquered something. By dinner time I am still feeling a bit off keel and not hungry at all, but I eat what I can and call the day a success. My first full day on chemotherapy is officially behind me. And now I know this is doable. I can handle this. And one small keyhole of light shines through the terrible darkness I had created in the cavern of my fear.

Staring Down the Beast

I HAVE MY FIRST DOSE of chemotherapy behind me. But I am still finding myself alternating between swimming in darkness and confusion and pumping myself up to go into battle. Based on my response to the first dose, I feel like I should be able to go back to work at least a few days a week. It might be a welcome distraction. When I am home I get really down and find myself fixating on bad thoughts. My director eventually calls me. I know he wants to know my game plan. I really have left them hanging. Am I quitting? Taking leave? Or will I be back Monday? He is nothing but supportive and even tells me, "I would completely understand if you never wanted to see another breast biopsy."

Hmmm. Never see another breast biopsy? The thought hadn't even crossed my mind. I still wanted to see my own biopsy in fact.

But the bigger question is really *what do I want to do with the rest of my life*, especially if it turns out to be shorter than I expected. I think about quitting my job and spending more time with my kids. I think about moving to the water somewhere and opening an art studio. *Would these changes bring me more happiness?* After mulling over many possibilities, changing my life does not seem like the right answer, at least for now. I chose the path I am on for a reason. About a month before I was diagnosed I vividly remember driving to work and experiencing this spooky feeling of something close to perfection—that scary realization that I have all the things I wanted at this stage in my life, and that meant I also had a lot to lose. And now here

I am faced with losing literally everything. So I decide I want to fight back and stay in the game. I will be back to work on Monday, I tell my director. I will take chemo-Wednesdays off and probably the day after to recover. But I will not be throwing in the towel. I still have work to do, damn it.

The next Monday, I timidly show myself again at work. Even though I feel the same physically, I am now a "sick person" walking the halls. I have just started chemotherapy but still have a full head of hair. Despite my still unscratched exterior, emotionally there is a mother lode of fear and sadness lying just beneath my surface. My colleagues and residents stop by to give me well wishes. One poor resident cries in my office and I find myself comforting her. This must be a big shock to the residents, many of whom are my age. People who go through medical school are supposed to study and treat diseases, not get them themselves. But I am an unsettling example for them that no one is immune.

It feels good to know people care about me so much, but I actually don't like it when other people cry for me. It makes me feel like they think I am going to die, even though I know they are probably just feeling my pain for going through this. But at this point I privately do think I am going to die of this, and I don't really want other people thinking so too. It's too early for that.

After I settle in for my first day back as my new cancer-ridden self I take a look at my first slide under the microscope. Ahhh . . . there is the world I love again, the work I am good at. The focus on something other than myself feels really good. I am quickly back in my diagnostic mode. I always thought about the newly diagnosed women to whom the slides I look at belong. I read their histories and imagine what it would be like to be them. But I always looked for reasons that made me different from them—oh, she has a strong family history or she must have ignored her symptoms—so that it could not actually be applicable to me. But now I know how it feels firsthand— the swirling black hole of the terrifying unknown opening before you when you hear the words, "It's cancer." Now I want to footnote each report for newly diagnosed women with a personal message.

> *FINAL DIAGNOSIS: Left breast, core needle biopsy: Invasive ductal carcinoma, Nottingham grade 2 . . . PS: So sorry, honey. Welcome to the club no one wants to join. Be strong, you will get through this. Survivors rule.*

Later I gather up the strength to take a look at my own biopsy. I am picturing a really blue tumor with big, dark nuclei gathered together in big cohesive sheets. These are the kinds of high-grade cancers I have seen melt away with chemotherapy. I look at the slide label and feel the strangeness of seeing my own name there. On the scope it goes. I peer into the eye pieces and take a look at my enemy. It is hideous. Ugly pink cells tearing their way through the tissue with complete disregard for the normal cellular boundaries. Not growing in sheets but in cords and single cells in a frighteningly infiltrative manner. They form abortive lumens filled with scant secretions, like they are attempting to make toxic lactational change. There is even an area where the malignant cells are nesting up with spaces forming around them, like they are trying to make their own vessels to feed themselves. The ugly bastards are even floating in lymphatic spaces, attempting to escape my breast altogether to wreak havoc in whatever other organ they can gain access to. And I see their precursors, the pre-invasive ductal carcinoma in situ, which is also really pleomorphic, scarring up formerly normal ducts so they are nearly unrecognizable. The biopsy of my lymph node was no better. The worst of the cancer was in there and had been there long enough to cause a lot of scarring.

Something had gone terribly wrong here. Some horrible mutation had occurred and sent these cells wildly out of control. This was not a well-behaved, slow growing cancer, this was a formidable enemy. I am amazed I could have been so unaware of this malignant creature growing inside me. Ironically, it was probably growing at the same time my sweet little son was also growing inside me (even more ironic is the fact that Henry's astrological sign is Cancer). I had read up on pregnancy-related cancers before all this, and the thought was that the raging hormones make breast tissue proliferate faster, giving it a chance to make cell division mistakes. And since your immune system is in "tolerate a pregnancy/parasite" mode, it may not kill off abnormal neoplastic cells that it normally would recognize and take care of before they grow out of control. And then with how swollen and lumpy lactational breasts are, there is not a great way to pick something up on self-exam. Like the perfect storm catching you unprepared.

This is all just a horrible mistake, I keep telling my cancer, like it is an unwanted child. *You will have to go. You were a horrible mistake.*

On Pregnancy and Ports

M AYBE IT IS BECAUSE I go through both experiences so close together, but getting chemotherapy reminds me a lot of being pregnant. Both states have a constant low-level nausea that is worse on an empty stomach. Both send waves of fatigue crashing over you so that sometimes it seems impossible to stay awake even though it is only seven thirty at night. Your hair gets thick and then falls out (although to a much milder degree after pregnancy!). You are not supposed to go in hot tubs or get deep tissue massages. Biologically your body is adjusting to a situation where you are host to a foreign invader in both pregnancy and cancer. Your immunity is compromised and you get sick easily. And people who see either your growing belly or your bald head offer you their chairs and treat you with a mix of fear and empathy. People send you flowers and fruit-of-the-month clubs and home-cooked meals when the times get tough. And in a way, going through cancer treatment is like a rebirth.

So strangely, some of this is feeling like familiar territory. And in some ways it is easier than pregnancy because I know I will never be at the stage where I have to haul around a bowling-ball-sized abdomen, waddle like a duck, and then push a watermelon out an orifice that seems *way* underequipped for the job. Instead I will get skinny and may be able to buy jeans in a size I haven't seen since high school—got to have *some* perks.

After my first few weeks of the Red Sunshine, I am scheduled to get a port placed. A port is basically a little device placed
under the skin that is threaded into the major vessels leading to
your heart. Instead of having to start an IV for each round of
chemotherapy, my nurse will just access my port with a special
modified IV needle and deliver the goods without burning up my
smaller peripheral veins. This all sounds good and easy, but what
I am really most excited about is *who* is going to place my port.
Dr. Hickman has to be in his eighties by now, but the nurses all
say that they never have a problem with the ports he places. He
is no ordinary surgeon. He basically *invented* the port (the earlier
version was called a Hickman line). He has come in and out of
retirement multiple times because he simply could not stay away
from the operating room for long (and he claims his wife didn't
like him hanging around the house.) So now he places ports in
a small operating room at the Seattle Cancer Care Alliance for
lucky patients like me, the vast majority of which I am sure are
oblivious to his fame.

Ryan and I show up for my 7:00 AM port-placement procedure, and a nurse gets me gowned up and puts a surgical cap on
me. I am eagerly waiting to meet "the man behind the port," and
he shows up right on time—a tall, long-fingered man dressed in
surgical blues with intelligent eyes and a well-creased face.

"Dr. Hickman, it is an honor!" I sit up and offer my hand to
shake. He looks quite pleased at this recognition. He has read
my chart and knows I am a pathologist, so he gives me a detailed
rundown about how the ports work and how exactly he will
place it, and he hands us an example port to play with. He tells
Ryan that he can join him in the operating room. Ryan is usually
quite squeamish but he actually takes him up on the offer. Dr.
Hickman gives me a bit of his history. He apparently was in the
first residency class at the University of Washington back in the
50s. Then he goes on to tell me the story of how he first came up
with the idea of using an indwelling central line.

"You see, the wife of a hospital VIP got cancer and needed chemotherapy. They couldn't get an IV started on her because she was . . . well, she was a large woman. So they called me in. And I said, ' why don't we put in a central line?' No one was doing that in this country so they all thought I was crazy. But it worked like a charm and she got her chemotherapy on schedule with fewer complications."

He leans toward me and feels around on my chest just below my collar bone.

"I think only a small-sized port will fit on you. It should be tucked in right down here a few inches below the collarbone. You won't even see it when you wear a regular shirt. I had a woman come in once with a wedding gown. A full length gown! And she told me 'now Dr Hickman, this is what I'll be wearing at my wedding and can we please have the port placed below the neckline.' I told her now *that* was a special request!"

I don't want to stop listening to his stories, but eventually it is time for me to climb up on the operating room table. I will be getting conscious sedation, like the kind you get when you have your wisdom teeth pulled and you feel like you were awake the whole time but you can't remember a thing. A big blue surgical drape is placed over me, and an assistant tells me to start watching the clock in the room. I try to concentrate on the minute hand, but the next thing I know the whole procedure is over and they are pulling the drape off. I look down and there is a small knob under the skin of my right chest with some fresh sutures to the right of it. Under my gown, where it sticks up slightly, it looks a bit like an accessory nipple, confused and floating upward toward my collarbone.

Overall, it does make chemotherapy easier. There is no missing a vein and leaving with bruised arms. It is a one shot deal. Although it is a bit odd to have someone ask you to lean your back against a chair so they can jam a large bore needle into your chest. It only stings for a second when the needle is placed, though. The real problem ends up being Henry's strange ability to find the port with his little fingers and give it a good squeeze whenever I am holding him on my right hip. Little port-pincher!

Fallout

WHEN ONE PERSON IS diagnosed with cancer, there is an emotional fallout that affects all those surrounding them. Everyone reacts differently and many are not sure exactly how to react. I try to give everyone a wide berth on this, recognizing that most people have no idea what to do in this situation.

I am sure my parents are terrified. I can't imagine watching my child go through this. I think my father, a German-born economist, has a view of cancer as a death sentence, something to bow your head down to, take your medicine, and wait in serious silence hoping for a cure. I can tell he is uncertain about what his supportive role is in this whole endeavor since he is usually my advice giver and this is an area where his expertise is less than mine.

My mother, always a pleaser, has impressed me with her positive "attack this thing" attitude. Helping take care of other people is definitely her area of expertise, and she has amazingly agreed to fly up from San Francisco every other week to come help out with the kids, meals, and life in general. My younger brother, Chris, is also at a bit of a loss. He lives in Seattle right now, having moved up here to help Ryan open his new business. He is also a pleaser, like my mom, but in this situation I think he really has no clue what exactly would please me. He volunteers to shave his head in solidarity. I beg him not to (one baldy is enough in the family) and so he settles for a really out-of-date crew cut. I feel the love.

And then there is Ryan. Ryan is a man of action. He likes to build and create things, like new businesses. He is competitive by nature, having been an Olympic-level rower, but is also incredibly good with people. I've never met anyone who didn't love his sense of humor and easy nature. He has dealt with hard times before, with the death of both his brother and father, and I think that at first he just felt in shock by the unfairness of yet another blow to someone he loves. But he has quickly come out of this mind-set. He is a survivor already. His mother is the same way. When times get tight, you *do* something about it and get through it without dwelling. He is self-sufficient and expects me to be as well.

One day I am lying in bed, crying—my mind playing out all sorts of end-game scenarios. Ryan is next to me but feels worlds away. He has just been talking about some future plan about what he wants to have done five years from now. I am torn up wondering how he can possibly think that far ahead into the future and so easily see me still with him.

I turn to him and ask tearfully, "Why aren't you more worried about me?"

"Look, I know that every day either of us could be killed in a car accident. But you can't live in fear of it."

It is true. And he does know this firsthand. Life can be snuffed out in an instant. But knowing you have a limited potential to make it to the next five years doesn't make it any easier to ignore my mortality. And a little empathy would really be nice. A little "My poor wife, I am so sorry you are going through this" would feel good. Or then would we *both* just be weeping messes?

My mother tells me that most men are not hard-wired for empathy. It is not an evolutionary advantage for a man to have empathy, but the women who traditionally take care of the infants and kids who scrape their knees and get sick, they need empathy to make sure the next generation continues.

When she brings this up one night at the dinner table I pipe in.

"Ryan has never felt sorry for anyone. When the kids or I are sick, all he wants to do is stay away from us so he doesn't catch it. I don't even get any sympathy for having cancer!" He answers back, "I am not sorry Kim has cancer, I just want to know what to *do* about it."

And what he *does* give is a strong show of support. He has decided to go with me to every chemotherapy appointment. It is our "chemo-date" on Wednesday afternoons. We will have lunch and then I will have a toxic cocktail, but he will be there to make me laugh and keep me company. He might fall asleep sitting in the big, puffy, marshmallow-like recliners that are arranged next to the bed. The whir of the IV is a bit mind-numbing, so I don't blame him and I don't mind. It is not entirely quiet for long here, with nurses and my favorite chaplain poking in all the time, always to talk to *me* about how *I* feel. Ryan is not used to me getting so much attention. We always joked about how "high maintenance" he is because he really likes to always have my full attention. Sitting at the dinner table sometimes I feel like I have three kids begging for my energy to focus on them. But here he is giving up his cherished workday, to sit bored out of his mind listening to me talk about my cancer or gossiping. And that is his way of standing by me.

Mothers and Daughters

I KNOW MY HAIR WILL be gone soon. It has been over three weeks since I started chemotherapy and I was expecting my "molting" to have already taken place. Over the last few weeks I have been secretly tugging on small fingers full of hair to test out how solidly anchored it is. And so far it has not budged a bit. I feel like I have not earned my wings or something since I don't have the classic chemohead. Finally today for the first time when I tug on a strand, it lets go easily. It is not falling out on its own yet, but it is just barely hanging onto its follicles. Here we go. Baldness awaits me.

This means I have to tell Maddy before she is left to wonder why her mom suddenly went skinhead. I don't want to make it a big ordeal. Small digestible pieces of information are all she needs. So instead of a big speech, I just stop her casually in the hallway and get down on one knee to look her in those big brown eyes.

"Hey Maddy, I have been meaning to tell you something," I start.

"Yeah Mom?" she replies. She likes it when I am looking right into her eyes on her level.

"My doctors found something in me that they need to fix. So they are giving me some medicine to help make it better. But the medicine is going to make Mommy's hair fall out for a while and might make me a little more tired or sick."

She looks at me as if she is taking this information in, so I continue.

"But my hair will grow back when I am finished taking the medicine," I add.

"Like grass?" she asks.

I instantly can see the image she sees of her mother's shiny bald head growing hair back like a chia pet. Grass gets mowed, and then it grows back. Ahh . . . the logic of childhood.

"Yes! Exactly like grass," I respond and wait for any more questions or negative reaction.

"OK!" she quips cheerfully and skips off down the hallway.

Now *that* went easier than I expected! Did she even get it? Everything is cool in that four-year-old mind as long as things will go back to normal at some point. This serves as a good reminder to me that it actually could happen. My hair *will* at some point grow back like grass and things *will* go back to some state of normalcy. *Thanks, Maddels.*

The next week I am driving her and a friend to a park for a playdate, and I hear Maddy tell her friend proudly, "My mom is going to lose all her hair and then it will grow back, like grass." The friend is clearly impressed—and so am I.

Now that things are starting to form a new routine, I am suddenly finding that life is getting pretty easy. My mother and Ryan's mother are alternating weeks that they come up to help with the kids and with cooking from Tuesday to Friday. And my colleagues at work all chipped in to get me a meal delivery service I use on the other days. I just have to sit back and take my medicine. I show up for wonderfully cooked organic meals. My taste buds are not the same as they used to be, but I am still eating. And just having someone else feed the rest of the family is a real treat. In the year before my diagnosis, Ryan was working a lot of nights and weekends at the new restaurant. I had a new baby, we had just started a fledgling high-maintenance business, and I was struggling to get my career off the ground. There was no time for myself. No time to sit back and relax. I felt like I was running around trying to make sure everyone and everything was taken care of. And now here I am being tended to and fed like I am the kid again. And I actually have time to meet with a trainer once a week, get acupuncture, go to yoga classes, and relax on my day off from work. The kids are bathed when I get home each day, happy as clams because they got to play with Grandma. The house is clean and dinner is ready. What more could a working woman ask for? At last I have a wife!

The grandmothers like the deal too, I think. They are spending so much quality time with the grandkids at a time when they are so rapidly changing. They go home for a week and when they come back, Henry has learned a new word or trick and Maddy is a little bit taller. I assure them that we will all survive if they need to skip a week, but they will have none of that. I know it is not easy on them traveling from California to Seattle every other week, leaving their jobs and lives and husbands on hold. My father doesn't really know how to feed himself anything but cheese and salami, so I guess I recognize his sacrifice too. He joins my mom on a few trips, but that actually means one more person for her to take care of. I think she really likes to feel needed, and I really do need her right now. So the deal stands and I relish every day of it. Moms rule.

Teamwork

RYAN AND I ARE sitting in the puffy, marshmallow-colored chairs in the infusion bay, chatting it up with nurse Cathy. Being a nurse is kind of like being a saint. A doctor diagnoses and prescribes, but a *nurse* is the one who really takes care of you when you are in need. When you are having a baby, it's your nurse who stays by you and makes sure you are getting your ice chips, receiving appropriate encouragement, and progressing along nicely. The doctor just whizzes in for the grand finale. When you get chemotherapy, you meet with your oncologist about once a month but you see your nurses constantly. I seem to alternate between three infusion nurses.

Sandy was my first. She really suits her name, with wavy sandy grey-blonde hair and sparkling eyes. She shares with me stories about her life about how she used to live on the beach in Cape Cod raising seven children, several of which were invited into her happiness by adoption. I imagine her as a young mother watching her brood have adventures on the beach on a hot summer day as she sips a homemade lemonade and digs her toes in the perfect sand. Now she and her husband take the grandkids out on their sailboat for adventures in the San Juan Islands. She exudes patience and peace and makes me calm just being near her.

Cathy was next. The minute she cruised into my room with her wavy auburn hair and easy smile, I knew we would be friends. She gives me recommendations on good smoothie recipes, her favorite yoga instructors, and where to get reiki massage. She asks me a lot of questions about what I do and what it is like to be experiencing things from the other end. She even shares with me the details of her struggle to have kids, and I think how lucky I am to have two kids of my own. I know it is her job to take care of me, but I think we would be friends if we met elsewhere as well.

And then there is Janine. She has short brown hair and fine color-rimmed glasses. She is no-nonsense. She looks you right in the eye when she talks to you and uses your name a lot in conversation. She pays attention to everything about you because you are her patient. She has raised two boys, who are now in their twenties, and you get the feeling that she taught them independence and efficiency. I feel in very capable hands with her.

So today is nurse Cathy's day and we are talking about some nut butter smoothie recipe. Ryan is practically asleep. The Red Sunshine is snaking its way up the tubing into my port as we socialize. Ryan sits up as he gets a phone call and excuses himself. He comes back and sits down.

"Who was it?" I ask at a pause in the conversation.

I see his eyes fill with tears and I am suddenly worried he is about to deliver bad news.

"Is everyone OK?" I ask.

He is having trouble answering.

Finally he gets out "That was Mike."

Mike is one of Ryan's oldest friends from college. They rowed together on the University of Washington (UW) varsity rowing team and later were pair partners on the United States National team. I met Mike the same day I met Ryan. I was a senior in college and very close to graduation. My girlfriends and I had just turned in our senior thesis papers and found ourselves for one of the first times in our college careers with nothing to do on a warm Sunday night in May of 1997. Some of my girlfriends were rowers and they knew the guys who were training on the national team from interacting at the boathouse. We decided to pick up some margarita mix and tequila and head off-campus to the house that a lot of the guys from the team stayed at. As we pulled up into the driveway, I saw some studly-looking men just backing out of the driveway. They saw that a carload full of co-eds had just arrived, and they quickly re-parked their car. Out walked Ryan and Mike, two six-foot-four handsome, tan blonde men. *Now, where had these guys been hiding my whole senior year?* I generally was a sucker for the goofy nerdy types, but this was like something out of a movie. We had a very innocent night of flirtation, margaritas, and playing pool, and I remember thinking *well that was fun but I'll probably never hear from them again. I start medical school in a few months and I am off to other things.* A few nights later Ryan left me a message on my campus phone asking if I remembered him (*umm . . . yes!*) and would I like to go to New York City to hear the Gypsy Kings play at a new restaurant in Soho?

Hell yes.

It was a double date with Mike and his date. We spent the rest of the summer falling in love, laughing hysterically, and kicking back in that beautiful time that is between one chapter and the next. The rest is history.

So Mike had been friends with Ryan since college, lived and rowed together afterwards, seen us as a couple from the beginning, was a groomsman at our wedding, and was still a regular in our lives now that he was the varsity coach for UW.

"Mike is having his varsity boat row on Opening Day with pink W's on their shirts . . . for you, for us . . . ," Ryan chokes.

"Oh my god." And I feel tears coming on as well. This was quite an honor. Every team proudly displays their team colors on their jerseys. The UW's are purple and gold and they have never *not* worn their team colors in a race. To change to pink was a big statement and a bold one for his first year as varsity coach. What a thing for a friend to do.

As the Opening Day races approach, I notice more of my hair falling out. I knew I was going to shave it off at some point but this timing gives me an idea. It is tradition for first year rowers at UW (or "grunties") to shave their heads before a big race. Ryan, Mike, and their friend Phil all did it. What if I had my head shaved at the boathouse the day before Opening Day? We call Mike and it is a done deal.

That Friday at work I start having second thoughts. I tug at my hair over and over to make extra sure that it really is falling out. Yes, whatever I grab hold of falls out, but I still have what appears to be a full head of hair. Do I really want to get rid of it all now instead of waiting until it is really patchy and pathetic looking? But from what I have read, I am on the brink of losing it all and people who don't shave it off first end up with a pillow full of hair one morning and then it goes in fistfulls. I don't really want to go through the clogged shower drains and the long good-byes. And for some reason, since the hair loss has taken longer than I expected (it has been four weeks since my first dose), I feel ready now to go for the full Monty. I should really look more the part of a chemotherapy patient by now.

I have already gone wig shopping and picked out a lovely chin-length dirty blonde named Erika. (Yes, I was intrigued to learn that wigs come with their own names like they are some sort of pet to be adopted.) And I have a few scarves in case I can't stand Erika sitting on my head all day like a dead squirrel. I tried her on for Maddy, and she told me I looked like Shaggy from Scooby Doo. I clearly need to learn a little about grooming Erika before she goes live. Henry on the other hand looked at me like I was definitely *not* the mother he knew and loved. He managed a slight lower lip quiver and then I got a smile when I pulled it off again to reveal my naturally limp hair. Erika may not be my new best friend after all. I will probably go with the scarf—maybe get some crazy pirate look going, or add some fruit on top for a tropical flare . . .

So today is the day. I walk over to the boat house after work and meet Ryan and the kids and some other friends who came for support (i.e., to see if I have a bumpy head under my hair.) Mike meets us in his office and tours us around first. He shows us the boats, the launch, the locker rooms, and the boat we will be riding on tomorrow to watch the races. Then we get to the workout room and he walks us up to the trophy case. Inside are countless trophies and plaques and, oddly, in one area of the display case there are a bunch of awful looking, poorly sewn, and lavishly decorated pillows.

"What are those?" I ask.

"These are the hair pillows," Mike explains.

"What? Hair pillows?" I ask the obvious question.

"Yes, hair pillows. Every year the freshmen who shave their heads make a class pillow stuffed with the shavings. Check out that one with the dreadlock tassels."

I look closer and see some of the pillows have tiny hairs poking through the fabric. Now this is some crazy sick stuff but funny. Why not bring a little humor to something like shaving your hair off? Too bad I won't have enough hair from my one head for a whole pillow. It takes a team for that kind of craftsmanship.

"And this is the captain's chair." Mike points to an oversized wooden chair with purple and gold leather covering.

"This is where *I* had my head shaved," says Ryan proudly. "Only the captain of the crew team can sit in this chair *except* when you are getting your head shaved as a freshman."

Mike shows us a picture of a young Ryan with a big smile and half of his hair gone. He is sitting in the very same Captain's chair.

At this point a small crowd of team members and my friends has gathered. Mike introduces me to some of his guys. They look so young and vital standing around casually in their skimpy unitards. One of them was diagnosed with Hodgkin's lymphoma last year and went through chemotherapy with the Red Sunshine as well. And here he is, a strong, robust athlete back in action. I am suddenly excited to shave my head. I'm like part of the team here. It is not a morbid sad affair or a going away party. It feels like it is for fun, for a statement, for an initiation.

"All right, are you ready?" Ryan seats me in the chair and I look out shyly at everyone. They look mostly curious if I will go through with it.

"Ready!" I pipe and look down quickly.

Ryan pulls out the electric hair clippers and places them against my head. Cameras flash. Maddy and her friends stop running around to watch. Ryan runs the shaver over my head in rows like he is mowing a lawn. I feel the vibrations against my skull and watch as my hair tumbles down in showers to the floor below me. I am so curious what my head will look like unveiled. Will it be bumpy and dented? And strangely, I am feeling liberated. No more bad hair days. No more money on highlights. This will be just me, raw and exposed.

Ryan trades the clippers for a shaver to get a closer crop. When he is done, I venture towards the mirror and take a long hard look at the new me. My head is not too bumpy. My eyes look really big now and I have a quiet toughness about me. I notice a mole I never knew I had. But all in all, it is not the end of the world by any measure. And, as Maddy said, it will grow back like grass someday.

I try out one of my scarves and have to figure out for the first time how to tie it so it stays. I am thinking about all the different colors and patterns I would like to go shopping for. We drive home with me staring at my reflection the whole way. Ryan keeps rubbing my head like I am a good luck charm. He tells me I look sexy. Who knew hair loss could spice up your sex life?

The next morning I proudly display a bright pink headscarf as I watch the men's team win their Opening Day race sporting their pink Ws. I feel like a celebrity as I cheer from the race launch. We even make the newspaper.

Thanks, Mike.

Life in the Short-Term

I AM A PLANNER. I make lists for the short-term items I need to get done and have always had a mental list of the things I want to have done in the long-term. I hate not knowing what is around the next bend in life and I do whatever possible to avoid uncertainty.

I remember when I was in high school, trying to decide what I wanted to do with my life. I was debating about pursuing something creative like marketing, advertising, or writing versus using my love of biology and knack for memorization to launch a career in science or medicine. After weighing what I thought were all the pluses and minuses, I based my decision on the idea that I could work really hard and probably do reasonably well on the medical/science track but it was much higher risk to go after a creative career because raw talent— not just hard work—would be required for success. What if I had no creative talent? Then I would risk complete failure. Better to stick to a path that has a clear track to run on without surprises. Better to play it safe. Don't get me wrong, I do occasionally relish a completely unscheduled day. I did backpack through Europe in my early twenties—but I always called to the city ahead for a room.

And I have to say that up until now, all has gone loosely as planned. There have been moments when the path veered off from my chosen direction. Relationships sure do have a way of not going according to plan. I remember vividly the day that I wanted my college boyfriend, my first real love, to take me back after a bad fight and he had coldly refused. *How could this be? Something I wanted so badly and planned for was simply not going to happen?* I remember my hand on the doorknob of his dorm room as I was about to leave both the room and the relationship and realizing that I was on the threshold of a chapter in my life that I was not expecting (a life without him). So instead of turning the knob, I crumpled to the ground in a humiliating heap of self-pity at the doormat. I had lost control of this situation and nothing I could do would make it successful. So I just could not bring myself to leave. He was unfazed by my soap opera antics and told me to get up and get out—which eventually I managed to do.

And I had learned that happiness does not necessarily come from hard work and success in your chosen path. Unlike many of my more clinically minded colleagues, I relished my first two years of medical school when I could bury myself in textbooks and discover the miraculous machinery that lives inside the human body. I liked the instant feedback I would get from exams—all the pats on the back for working hard and doing well. But then, when it came time to rotate through the wards, I was shocked at how uncomfortable I was not knowing what was wrong with a patient and how my schedule was now completely controlled by my superiors. I was deprived of sleep and at the bottom of the food chain. I was dating Ryan, and he had moved across the country from New York to Seattle after his father died. I could not get him to visit me enough, and I was afraid of losing him because I couldn't follow him. And to top it all off I was realizing that I actually didn't like clinical medicine at all. I didn't like the tapping and poking and educated guesswork. I didn't like the thinking on your feet and constant prescribing. I dreaded going to the hospital for tedious rounds where we roused sleepy patients before sunrise to stick cold stethoscopes under their robes and ask them if they had passed gas overnight. The best part was the personalities I encountered in the patients I met, but the actual *work* of clinical medicine left me feeling like I was missing the point that my co-students all had finally found. I wanted to go back to studying. Return to living in my own imaginary world. I was realizing with panic that my grand plan was not going to make me happy after all. What was I to do, jump ship after all this investment? Get a messy divorce from my career?

But just when it felt like I had really lost my vision, I managed to find my way out of the confusion. One sweltering summer day during my medicine rotation at a non-air-conditioned city hospital in Spanish Harlem, I had been assigned to a beautiful young female exchange student who recently arrived from Africa. She was suffering from fatigue and high fevers, and our team had not been able to figure out quite what was wrong. Top in our differential diagnosis was malaria. Hence, I was sent to draw her blood so the lab could search it for the tiny ring-shaped parasites. I hand delivered the small tube of blood to the lab, and they directed me to a pathologist working in the back. She asked if I wanted to look at the blood myself, and I thought *why not?*

When I looked into the microscope and saw the field of disc-shaped red cells spread out before me, I dove right in. I searched for parasites with fervor, mistaking tiny round platelets at first as the bugs, comparing photos in a glossy paged textbook to what I was seeing. This was not like histology class where we just had to identify what something was. This was a visual mystery and I was looking for clues. *This* was exciting. We never did find a malaria parasite in that blood smear. It turned out she had Black Fever after all but later, on my surgery rotation, I found myself following specimens out of the operating room to the lab. What was this strange five-pound ovarian mass? Only the microscope could tell me. I had found my path again and did not have to jump ship. The controls were regained. I applied and was accepted to a pathology residency in Seattle, Ryan proposed, and my version of the fairytale continued.

And now here I am with the thing most vital to continue my story as planned being threatened—my future. The concept that my story could actually have a premature ending had actually occurred to me before. In fact, it used to cause me actual physical panic. My first year of medical school, when I just started learning about all the horrible diseases that could ravage the human body, I began the classic medical student paranoia believing that every headache was a brain tumor and every skipped heart beat was the start of a lethal arrhythmia.

One day on a plane ride across the country to visit Ryan, my heart did skip a beat and then literally began pounding in my chest. I started breathing fast and sweating. I was twenty-four years old and suffering a heart attack, and I was trapped on an airplane with no one to help me! I tried to calm down, but I kept checking my pulse, which of course made it only race faster. The flight attendant gave me a cold washcloth and told me to put my head between my knees. I felt completely out of control. A tightness gripped my throat. The poor man next to me recognized that I was having a panic attack because his wife had recently been diagnosed with them. It didn't help to hear him explain this to me because what I was feeling was *way* too physical to be caused by something mental. Eventually I calmed down, but I walked off that plane terrified of it happening again, which, of course, it did. In a crowded lecture hall, on a busy subway, at the movies—my ears would ring, my heart would pound, and my vision would blur with strange colorful auras. Ryan thought I was going crazy, so I tried not to talk about what was going on and suffered in private.

What was wrong with me? I went to the campus clinic and told the doctor there that my heart sometimes would pound, minimizing all the stranger details. The doctor told me that I was having premature ventricular contractions (PVCs), which are harmless skipped heartbeats that are followed by a stronger beat to make up for the skipped one. This might have calmed me some during that initial plane ride, but I was already in a vicious cycle of panic, so it didn't help much. The medical school psychiatrist told me to relax and maybe try having a glass of wine at night, or to try Prozac. *Drugs and alcohol? This was his recommendation to a young future physician who was clearly dying of something or other?* This was all quite unsatisfactory to me. I began to fixate on this intense fear of death and the panic, imagining all sorts of endgame scenarios (this was a time when an active imagination actually can do harm!). I was depressed and panicked, all at the same time.

I remember around this time an encounter with my mother that really put the first crack in the wall of fear I had been so busy building. I was on vacation with my family and my mother and I had gone on a bike ride to a lunch spot next to a lake. I had been quiet, living in my inner world of fear. As I sat there at the picnic table and looked out at the vastness of the placid water of the lake, I suddenly felt gripped by emptiness and I unexpectedly burst into tears. My mother was confused at this outburst of emotion.

"My God, Kim, what is *wrong?*" she asked, concerned.

I dropped my head into my hands dramatically.

"What if I die?!" I blurted out between sobs.

She waited until I lifted my head. Then she looked me right in the eyes and said, very matter-of-factly, "Then you die. It's not the end of the world."

This was an absolute shock coming from my super-sensitive mother who cries when she hears bagpipes playing and has empathy for everything from a mouse to a terrorist.

She also told me I must be hormonal, because to my mother everything in life is related to your hormones. But her uncharacteristically blunt answer to my question smacked me across the face like a hard slap. She did not try to calm me and claim that I wouldn't die. She just stated the facts: if you die, you die—period, end of story. No use being all dramatic about the possibility. I began to realize that what was gripping me so tightly was just a *fear* of death, not death itself. And a fear is something that I could control, yes?

Gradually, I started to educate myself about panic attacks, and the more I learned, the less afraid I became. Eventually, I learned to control my symptoms when they first began and they magically disappeared over the course of the year. I was back in control, and I felt stronger from the experience.

Now here I was again facing both an unexpectedly terrible twist of fate and that raw fear of the unknown that had resurfaced—ahhh ... the piercing beauty of the unexpected. What sort of trial will this be? I try to keep my spirits up, telling myself that this too will make me stronger. But every time I look at my children or my husband, I think of them having to deal with my death. What a horrible thing that would be for them to go through. And selfishly *I* want to be a part of their future. *I* want to be the one who gives my kids relationship or career advice. *I* want to be the one growing old with Ryan. It is *my* future, and it crushes me to think I might not be there for it.

I find myself wanting everything in fast-forward. I suddenly want to move to our dream house *now*. Ryan tries to reason with me. It is not a good time to move in the middle of all this, he tells me—but the feeling of urgency grows. I really want to leave this house and start over somewhere else—*now*. I know secretly I really just want to make sure I see at least part of the next chapter of our lives. I get angry at Ryan when he tells me we need to wait three or four years until his business is doing better and the housing market has recovered. This sets me in a tailspin. I can't even *think* about three or four years from now; how dare he even *talk* to me about three or four years from now. My whole life has been foreshortened, telescoped back on itself so that all I can really see is the here and now and the future is something completely unattainable. I cry myself to sleep that night and leave Ryan confused and bewildered.

I continue to have the "poor me's" the next day. That night we are meeting up with some friends for one of my first dinners out since the diagnosis. We get to the restaurant, and my friend Jessica starts earnestly asking me questions and offering support. She has just had her third child. He is the same age as Henry. She is six feet tall and beautiful. Her skin is glowing with youthful energy.

Everyone is poured a glass of wine except me. We are eating Indian food and everyone orders it spicy except me. I start to get that feeling like I'm the different kid in grade school, the loner with the funny haircut. Jessica tries to make contact with me, asking me questions about how I am feeling, how I am dealing, what is next. I am answering, but I am also feeling a jealousy rise inside of me for the first time. I am jealous of her vitality, of her health, and her youth. I am jealous that she won't have to go through menopause at thirty three years old. I am jealous that she doesn't have to worry about not seeing her kids grow up. I am jealous that she is drinking wine and ordering dessert, while suddenly I am a fragile, sober, cancer-riddled creature. I am tired by the end of the meal and ask Ryan to take me home a bit early.

Of course, of course—chemo girl needs her rest.

I am still feeling jealous and isolated the next morning, when Jessica and Claudia join us at our house for brunch. It is funny how you can feel so insular even though you are trying to surround your-self with people. But brunch goes as planned. Our kids are all play-ing happily together. Then my friends call me into the dining room. Spread across the table is a giant poster covered with photographs. I look down at it confused at first, and then I see the images of many familiar faces looking back at me. There is my friend from high school and college, Joanna, with her husband in London in front of the XOXO tower. There is Rochelle with a pearl necklace crossed in an X. People I haven't seen in years are holding up paper cutouts of Xs and Os. And there in the center is Ryan with a laughing Maddy and an in-motion Henry on his lap—my sun in this solar system of support.

I completely lose it. Seeing all those people holding up signs for me, cheering me on, feels so overwhelmingly powerful. I unleash the floodgates and the tears pour forth. I hug Jessica and Claudia and sob and sob until my shoulders shake. My jealousy evaporates and suddenly I feel like the luckiest person alive.

Religious Pressures

I'VE GOT ABOUT TWO months of therapy under my belt. I walk into the Land of Infusion like a pro now, strutting to my chemo bay, silk scarf tied in a crafty knot. I feel like Norm walking into Cheers as I greet my favorite nurses and receptionists. We know where the snacks and drinks for patients are stashed, and we stop there to stock up before I am chained up for my session of Red Sunshine. Ryan is rummaging through a drawer of Lorna Doones (why are they only found in hospitals or at blood donation drives now?) and NutriGrain bars, and I am grabbing two bottles of water when in waltzes my favorite chaplain.

"Hey you guys!" she says enthusiastically. She has a way of making you feel like she has been just waiting to see you for ages and ages. She has a big turquoise necklace on with matching earrings and of course is also sporting that heavenly twinkle in her eyes.

"Hi Deborah!" I am always just as excited to see her. We hug and then she leans back against the countertop ready to delve into conversation.

"What have you guys been up to?" We have not seen her in a few sessions. We catch her up on a whole lot of nothings.

Then she breaks into the question I had been waiting for her to ask since we met on my first day here.

"So I've been meaning to ask you guys what religion you practice." She tries to be casual, but I can tell she sees this as a nonthreatening place to bring this up—the snack room instead of trapped in my chemo bay.

"Ummm, well. My parents were raised Catholic and Ryan grew up going to a Lutheran church," I begin honestly. My parents *were* both raised good Catholics, complete with guilt and sin and first communion. My father was an altar boy at his local church back in Germany, where he grew up. My mother and her two sisters wore gloves and hats to their Whittier, California, church shepherded by their hardworking blue-collar parents. But then they left home and came of age in the 1960s and my mother found more meaning marching on the California state capitol and my father preferred economic modeling and chasing the girls in super-miniskirts instead of attending Sunday mass. When I was born, in 1974, they figured they would be progressive and not stifle me by choosing a particular religion to raise me with. We celebrated commercial Christmases and Easter bunny Easters but only went to church when my grandmother was in town. By their logic, I would eventually find my own religion if I needed to—but I never did. It is hard to feel like you are missing something if you never knew you needed it in the first place. In fact, if anything, I developed an intellectual fear of religion. It just seemed so intense and exclusive since everyone belonged to their own club that had their own initiation rites and ceremonies. And weren't the majority of history's wars related to disagreements about the best religion anyway? How could one religion be right and the others wrong?

And so I became an optimistic atheist. I liked the idea that we were just specks on a planet made of rock and molten lava and that everything around us was crafted by nature's discovered and undiscovered laws. Nature rocked. Why did the powerful balls of gas we call stars have to be made by someone in white robes? The forces of nature seemed much bigger than that. I figured we are all just sophisticated animals that bring meaning to our lives so that we can be more satisfied creatures. There was no man steering the wheel of the never-ending universe—it simply existed as a magnificent entity, just like we each exist as smaller magnificent entities spinning in our own little orbits.

Ryan's family is definitely more religious than mine. When Ryan's brother died they found a lot of strength from their church. It helped bring meaning to something that seemed so utterly meaningless. But Ryan wasn't particularly drawn to go to church at the time I met him. In fact, he didn't really talk about religion at all. He was a rower on the U.S. National Team and was more concerned with his rowing erg scores than if God was angry that he wasn't going to church every Sunday. But his family clearly cared about religion, and when it came time for us to get married, it seemed only fair that his youth pastor do the honors for us, since I had no religious ties. He was a young enthusiastic man with a modern vision of life and church, but I was still a bit surprised when he delivered a sermon at our outdoor vineyard wedding full of both good words and lots of references to the son of God. I remember my Jewish uncle, Don, coming up to me afterwards and saying, "Kimmy, I didn't know you invited the J-man to your wedding!"

"I didn't, Ryan did," I replied laughing.

And when my kids were born I kept waiting for the requests for baptisms but they respectfully never came or perhaps were performed in secret. Other people's beliefs were fine with me. I would never want to take away what gave some meaning to someone else's life. But don't try and sell it to me. Leave me to create my own meaningful universe.

And so, now that my favorite chaplain is waiting for me to elaborate on my religious beliefs, I am scared to tell her what I really think about the beliefs I know bring meaning to her life. And selfishly I want her to like me and to still visit my heathen sickbed.

"But . . . I wasn't really raised with much religion. Ryan is Lutheran," I repeat.

She isn't fazed. I remember her telling me she is married to a scientist.

"So what keeps you going? What do you believe in?" she asks with genuine curiosity.

"Well, I believe in the forces of the universe." I attempt to explain, but it sounds like I am in some sort of Star Trek cult.

"I mean, I feel like there is an energy out there and that we can create meaning from it all." I am not sure I am doing a good job explaining this to her and I don't want to shock her or Ryan with any atheist sentiments.

"So do you believe in a Heaven?" She asks point blank.

"Ummm . . . Do I think there is a shiny place where we look down from the clouds on the world below? No. But I'd like to think that the essence of our spirit lives on in some way. That it can't be lost because energy is never wasted, only transformed." I bring in the old law of conservation of energy. She seems to like this idea and we move on.

But I know that what I really believe is that when we die, our bodies become fuel for the creatures living in the earth, which feed other creatures, and on and on up the food chain. We get recycled like everything on Earth. What happens to the energy that makes up what we call our spirit is a bit more of an open question. The unique combination of brain connections that make up my mind won't likely be recreated, but I'd like to think it is recycled in some way. And although it sure sounds nice, I don't think I will be watching from heaven as the same being I am today. We are just creatures living on a planet and we will all die at some point. No escaping that—we *all* get to die some day. We can only hope for a good run this time around. I've always felt this pressure to make the most of life because of this belief. No waiting for anything in Heaven—do it *now*. I guess that is what keeps me going.

Just a Little Complementary Medicine

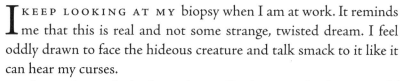

I KEEP LOOKING AT MY biopsy when I am at work. It reminds me that this is real and not some strange, twisted dream. I feel oddly drawn to face the hideous creature and talk smack to it like it can hear my curses.

I am going to absolutely crush *you. You have* no idea *how powerful I am,* I tell it to give myself strength.

One day at work after distracting myself with another cancer smack-down, I have an idea. I take a photo of my biopsy and label the image file "responder" (as in responder to chemotherapy). I know my best shot at long-term survival is to be in that lucky 40–50 percent that gets a complete pathologic response to chemotherapy—no cell left behind. It is all about my response to chemotherapy, and I *will* be a responder.

I print out a copy of the image on my printer. Despite my optimistic atheism, I feel the need to call on a higher power to get rid of this hideous beast. I may not have a religion to help me out, but I do feel the need for some form of spiritual healing. So I am going to try a little unconventional therapy to complement my chemotherapy.

I am going to do some magic . . .

I call my friend Claudia and tell her I want her to help me do a magical ceremony (as I try not to laugh). She is all over it. A few days later she shows up after dinner at my house with books on magic spells, candles, crystals, and other trinkets. She has studied up on the topic (this is my lawyer friend, not some pot-smoking flower child) and is prepared to lead us in a healing ritual. My mother is also in town and is totally game. None of us have done anything like this before. We giggle excitedly as we read about what we are supposed to do. We feel like a bunch of schoolgirls preparing for a secret society induction ceremony—some Ya-Ya sisterhood of witchcraft. I am suddenly wondering if we can take this seriously. Ryan decides to hide in the bedroom so he doesn't have to watch. I see our Catholic au pair creeping around and then escaping out the back door, probably in fear of her bizarre host mom.

We prepare three bowls, one with beads and a thread, one with a needle and a crystal, and one with the printout of my tumor. We bundle up with blankets and set up a bunch of candles on the cement patio outside. It is a clear, cold night with a decent wind. But the stars are so poignantly bright and the surrounding dark silhouettes of the trees so enchanting that we simply must have this setting to conduct the magic of course. We put on a CD of Hindu chanting that my mother's friend had given me. The magic had to like this!

Claudia picks up a piece of sidewalk chalk from my daughter's collection and draws a big circle on the cement. We have to repeat some chant about the circle as we walk around it, then step inside it and sit down. We state our intentions to the energy of the universe. I have to say out loud to the stars that we intend to heal my cancer so that it never returns. This is hard to do with a straight face. But Claudia is completely serious. She has warned us of the danger of not phrasing the intentions carefully, because saying something simple like "I want the cancer to be gone," might be misinterpreted and *you* could be gone along with the cancer. So I try to be very specific. My mom and I really want to giggle—I can see it in her eyes.

Clearly we are not experts at this. We keep having to refer to the book, the candles keep blowing out, and my dog keeps walking right through the middle of the sacred space. But we are having fun, and it feels good to be banded together against my enemy. We had decided to do some ceremony to energize the crystal with our intentions. We wanted to prick our fingers with the needle and each place a tiny drop of our blood on it. But either the needle is too dull and we cannot "break the circle" to go get something sharper, or we are just too timid with our needle sticks to draw blood. So we decide to each kiss the crystal and say a blessing on it (sissies!). Then I hold it up to the sky and say something about my intentions again. Next, we take turns stringing a bead on the thread, saying a healing chant each time, to make a power necklace. Again, technical difficulties arise because the holes in the beads are a little snug for the caliber of thread we have, so after some struggles we stop at seven beads, arguing that it is a lucky number.

Before we can get to the last magical task, the background music suddenly changes from the mystical chanting to a loud Dave Mathews CD that does not jive at all with the magic. Do we risk breaking the circle, which Claudia tells us is a big no-no, to reset the stereo and the magical mood? We decide we simply cannot risk it and proceed with Dave wailing around us.

Now for the part I have been waiting for. I unfold the printout of my cancer and take a good look at it. Then I strike a match in between gusts of wind, light the edges of the paper and place it back in the bowl. We all watch the image of my cancerous cells shrivel into slow black curls and then to ashes. I smile and feel truly powerful over my cancer for the first time since my diagnosis. *This is what's in store for you, you bastard! You think you can scare me! How do you like these intentions?*

We say some words that release the circle and then pack up. The sisterhood has spoken. I thank my cohorts, and we all go off to our beds.

The next day my daughter is playing outside and she sees the big chalk circle on the ground next to her playhouse.

"What's this?" she asks, a clever little observer. "This circle wasn't here yesterday."

"Maybe it's magic," I reply.

Yes, your professional mother is doing magic in the backyard while you sleep under your Hello Kitty bedspread. I doubt there is any evidence-based medicine supporting this!

Meltdown

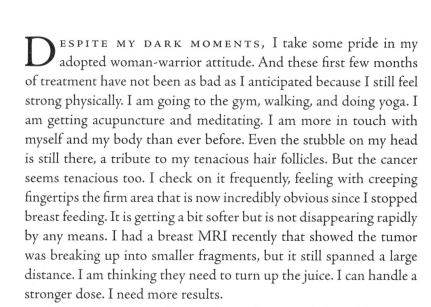

DESPITE MY DARK MOMENTS, I take some pride in my adopted woman-warrior attitude. And these first few months of treatment have not been as bad as I anticipated because I still feel strong physically. I am going to the gym, walking, and doing yoga. I am getting acupuncture and meditating. I am more in touch with myself and my body than ever before. Even the stubble on my head is still there, a tribute to my tenacious hair follicles. But the cancer seems tenacious too. I check on it frequently, feeling with creeping fingertips the firm area that is now incredibly obvious since I stopped breast feeding. It is getting a bit softer but is not disappearing rapidly by any means. I had a breast MRI recently that showed the tumor was breaking up into smaller fragments, but it still spanned a large distance. I am thinking they need to turn up the juice. I can handle a stronger dose. I need more results.

Then it starts to catch up with me. On my eighth weekly visit to the infusion ward I am upbeat, sitting in my infusion chair, feeling like a pro.

In walks my nurse, Sandy, with a real shocker, "So, your neutrophils are just below our usual cutoff to give you chemo."

"What?!" I balk. "They were normal last week." I feel like a kid used to getting A's now receiving my first D+. I am crestfallen. *What did I do wrong?* Then I remember one night last week I forgot to take my neutrophil-raising G-CSF shot ("G" shot for short) because I fell asleep early. That must be it. I confess my sin to Sandy, and she says she will contact my doctor to see if she can give me chemotherapy anyway. She leaves Ryan and me alone in our disbelief.

When she finally pokes her head back in she says "Hold up your right hand for me."

Confused, I raise my right hand.

"Now repeat after me. I, Kim Allison, promise to take all of my 'G' shots as directed."

I repeat the mantra—of course I will, of course.

"OK, Dr. Ellis says we can go ahead with the Adriamycin, but hold the oral Cytoxan for the week."

I am thrilled. Maybe I am becoming an addict, because I need my Red Sunshine now like a junkie. I know it makes me feel a little crappy, but mentally I feel like it is infusing me with hope and power. It is my best chance at survival, and I need every drop despite its toxic nature. I watch with a smile on my face as the ribbon of red fluid flows through the plastic tubing towards my port—ahhhh . . . I even think I can feel the cancer burn in response. I picture it shrinking in fear from the blinding light of the red sun I am unleashing.

The next week I take all my "G" shots. But even the best of neutrophil counts can't protect me from the nasty virus I end up catching from my kids. Both Madeline and Henry had been down for the count with weepy eyes, runny noses, and hacking coughs. And it is nearly impossible to hold a curious ten-month-old and not catch whatever germs they are serving up to you as they wipe their nose and then try to stick their tiny fingers in every orifice in your face. Realistically, I can't Purell my noggin.

We are headed out to our cabin in the mountains for Memorial Day weekend with friends, and I am feeling a sore throat coming on with a sense of doom. By the end of the weekend, I can't swallow without serious pain, can't sleep because of frequent coughing fits, and can barely get off the couch. I am so tired that I feel like I am becoming a faded version of myself. I try to help out or sit at dinner but I am not really there. I am just enduring, making myself intentionally numb. I want the time to pass and to be through this, but it feels like it will never end.

I have a doctor's appointment before I am scheduled to get chemo, the day after we get back. I have to wear a mask in the waiting room to protect all the other poor souls with weak immune systems sitting near me. Dr. Ellis takes one look at me and tells me to go home and rest. No chemo for me this week. I am not disappointed because I feel so awful. I know I need to get over this virus and chemo would not help with that—just a brief vacation from my sunshine.

The next week I sleep a lot. I have never liked naps, always finding myself so disoriented when I wake up, but now I cannot stay awake much at all during the day. I manage to make it to work one morning, but that is all I can handle. My cold starts to get better but then I start to get awful abdominal cramps. *What is going on? Colds don't transform into abdominal pain.* Then I realize I am getting my period—my first one in almost two years because I was pregnant and then breast feeding. I had nearly forgotten what it was, the pains of the monthly womanly curse! Here I thought I was coming down with some sort of abdominal emergency and it was just something women endure on a regular basis—what a wimp. But this is at least something I can treat with Advil and chocolate for once. Man, I thought I was supposed to be in menopause . . .

Chemo Wednesday rolls around again, and I feel weakened but recouped and ready to continue my fight. My mother-in-law, Gail, comes with me because Ryan is out of town. We are sitting waiting to see Dr. Ellis after having my labs drawn. One of the research coordinators comes over to me and asks me if I have been taking all of my "G" shots.

"Yes, every one," I answer raising my hackles. "Why, what is my neutrophil count?"

"Well, I'll wait for Dr. Ellis to go over it with you," she answers evasively.

"What do you mean? What is it?" I am pissed now and I have a bad feeling about this. *I can't miss chemo again. I can't get so off-track. I need to get all my therapy. How am I suddenly not able to withstand therapy? Will I not be able to finish?* I look out the vast windows in the waiting area that overlook Lake Union and watch a sea plane take off. I want to be on it, flying away from all of this to some remote location where nothing bad can happen.

Dr. Ellis suddenly appears in the waiting room area with a printout of my labs.

"What *are* you doing?" she asks me sarcastically and points to the place on the printout of my labs that has my neutrophil count. I stare at it in disbelief. Normal neutrophil counts are above 2.0 thousand/ml. They hold chemo if they are below 1.5. Last week mine was 1.66. This week it was 0.08—almost zero, the very bottom, with no chemo last week. My other labs looked awful as well.

"You've bottomed out, honey," she said. "But you don't look toxic so I'm going to send you home on antibiotics. Any fevers and I want you back here immediately."

I try hard not to cry. I don't really know what this means—if I can bounce back from this easily, or if I am going to be hospitalized. But I am terrified and disappointed.

All I can say is "Bummer."

Really professional.

And with that the tears come. My oncologist assures me that it is a normal reaction. *Great, I am having a normal reaction to abnormal labs.* She also assures me that the low counts are due to the chemo that was given two weeks ago, not because I couldn't bounce back anymore.

"I was beginning to wonder if you were an iron woman," she added, which just made the iron woman cry harder. My mother-in-law doesn't know what to do with me. I stare off into the distance for a while at the dreary Seattle weather. It is June and still rainy, cold, and shitty as February out. At least it matched my mood. We leave with a prescription for heavy hitter antibiotics to keep any bugs within me at bay while my defenses are gone and instructions to "continue my normal activities." Like in a bubble you mean? No Red Sunshine for the *second* week. The world feels like it is turning off axis.

But I remind myself that being so close to toxic must also mean destruction for the cancer. It must be melting with the toxic sunshine, unable to divide, shriveling on the vine. I just hope the rest of me doesn't do the same in the process. I go home and sleep, dreaming toxic dreams.

Rejuvenation

THE WEEK AFTER MY toxic meltdown I am planning to go with Ryan to Maui for a six-day getaway to celebrate our seventh wedding anniversary. The plan is to go without kids for our first long trip ever. I have been trying hard not to think about it. I don't want to get too excited and then have to cancel because of my ailing health. I made Ryan buy travel insurance, which he thought was a total waste because what could possibly go wrong? Plus, I was a little scared to travel. To get on an airplane full of people and their breath circulating in that stale recycled air, and to go to a moist tropical environment with lots of different exotic bugs to catch—I shouldn't go, it's too risky.

"People in Hawaii get cancer too, Kim, you know. And they get treated there," Ryan tells me.

He is right, but I still don't want to get my hopes up too much for the trip or for my neutrophils. I have had too many recent disappointments.

After a week of taking "G" shots and lots of visualizing of neutrophils pouring out of my bone marrow, I do manage to get my counts up to 2.0 and greet my old friend Mr. Red Sunshine again, with pleasure. I start to get hopeful again and I am happy I can board that airplane and go to Maui while I am fighting, not convalescing.

No one is coughing on the airplane and I keep the mask I brought in my bag and bravely breathe the recycled air. I am feeling slightly less fragile. When I get off the plane the air is warm and encompasses me like an embrace. I sink into the relaxed island aura with relief. The beach feels softer than I remember and the lava rocks darker and rich with heat. The first night the sun is setting in a cloudy sky but breaks through in thin slices, leaking thin showers of gold onto patches of the ocean. This is peace.

Early our first morning there, Ryan and I go for a long walk on the beachside path that winds past resorts and rocky cliffs. He decides to jog back and I am content to wander the path at my own pace, no longer trying to keep up with his long legs and strong heart. I watch a little white bird with a long beak and skinny legs walk on top of the bushes looking for snacks. I watch kids on boogie boards already out laughing in the waves. I watch an old couple getting ready to go for their morning ocean swim. I want to be them. I want to live to see that day when I am old and withered but still going for an ocean swim.

I climb down off the path onto a landing of lava rocks by the water and look out at the ocean. The vastness of it suddenly takes my breath away and makes me feel small. I can feel the energy of the world around me pulling with the waves and the wind. I want to be a part of it. I want to stay a part of this world so badly. I feel tears coming to the surface of myself and a wave of emotion surging from me. I turn toward the edge of the rocks, and I see something rolling gently in the water. I think at first it is a dead seal, with its rounded back tossing around in the waves—an omen of my own death. Then a tiny wise old head peaks up from the water in front of the body, and I realize it is a sea turtle. It turns to me and looks right at me as if I had asked it a question. Then it opens its mouth as if to say, "Don't worry. You will live long like the sea turtle." I smile through my tears. *Thank you,* I nod.

The rest of the trip I am at peace, maybe because of that encounter by the sea—but definitely also because Ryan and I are on our first long vacation together without children. For the first time I feel no guilt about leaving our offspring behind, and I am fully willing to focus on myself and our marriage. Luxuries like lounging poolside without interruption, having a full conversation, reading a novel, and sleeping whenever tired were on the short list of most missed tasks. There was the romance of eating out every meal and well, there was the romance. We left more in love and rejuvenated and vowed to return more regularly for "grown-up" vacation time.

The next time my labs are drawn pre-chemo, my neutrophils are sky high. I think my oncologist should prescribe me more vacation time.

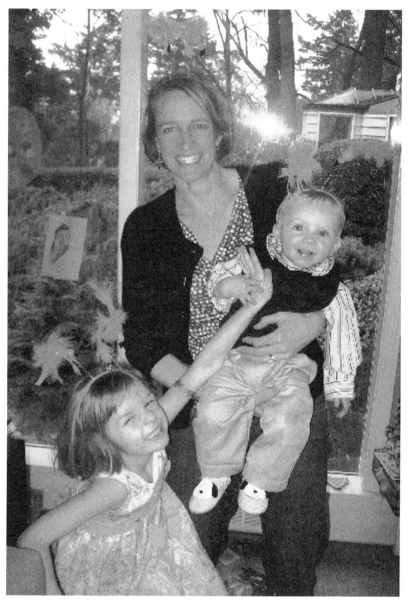

Life right before diagnosis with my two crazy kids: Maddy, age 4, and Henry, 7 months.

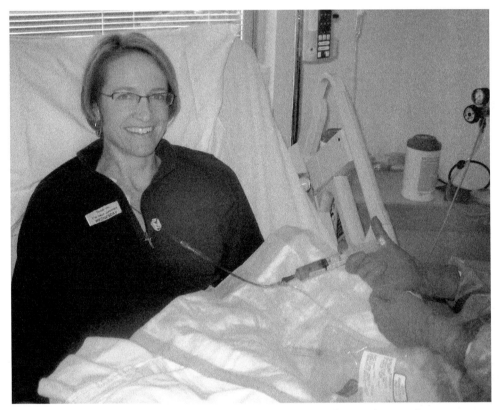

First dose of Red Sunshine. I'm only smiling because I am happy for it to be over!

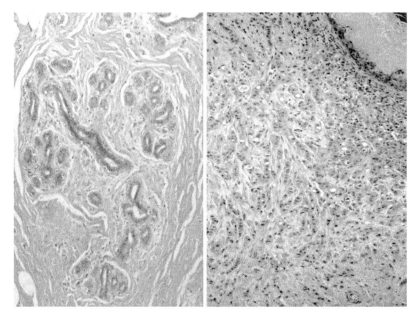

*Microscopic images of normal breast tissue (on the left)
and my cancer (on the right).*

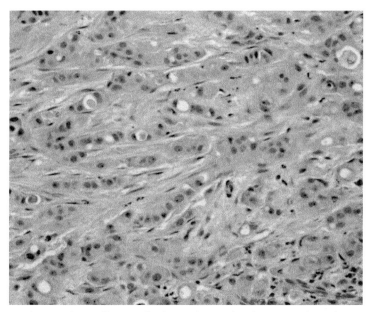

*The naughty cells gone bad, up close. They have no idea what
they are in for…*

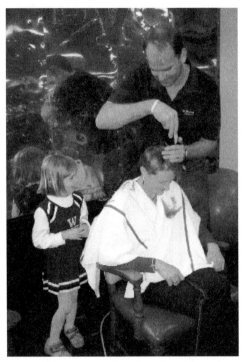

Ryan shaving my head at the University of Washington Boat House with Maddy looking on.

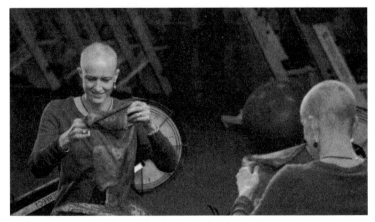

First look at the bald head!

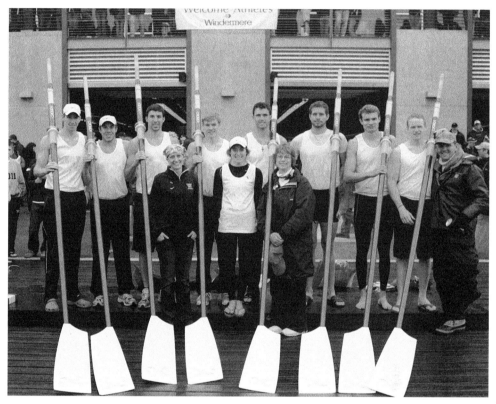

Opening Day with the University of Washington crew team (note the pink "W's" on their jerseys). Coach and friend, Michael Callahan, is pictured on the right.

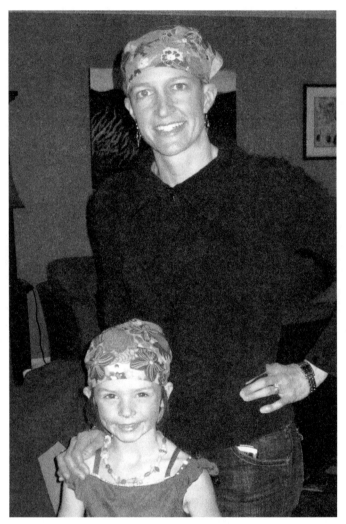

Mother and daughter modeling matching cancer-fashion.

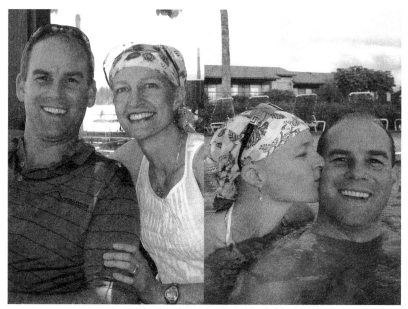

Ryan and I enjoy some time alone on vacation.

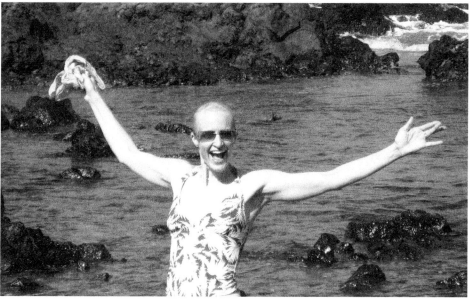

The bald head revealed.

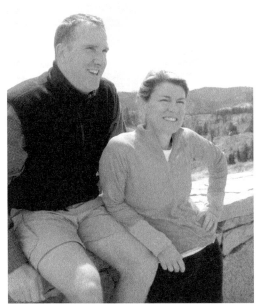

Claudia (my "nutrition guru") and her husband Chapin.

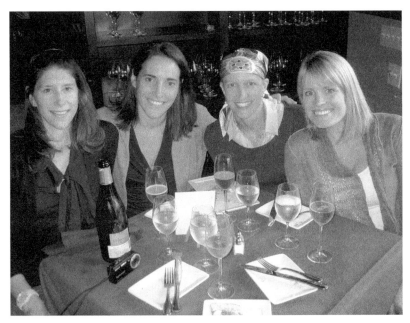

High school friends Joanna (my "international guru"), Naomi (my "check on my parents guru"), and Katie.

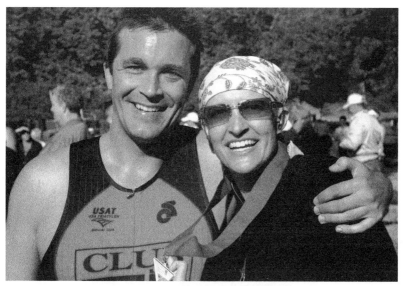

My brother, Chris, at his triathlon.

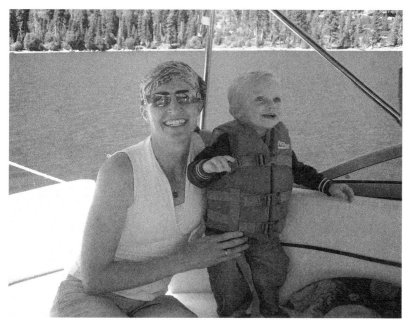

Lake Tahoe, California mid-chemotherapy.

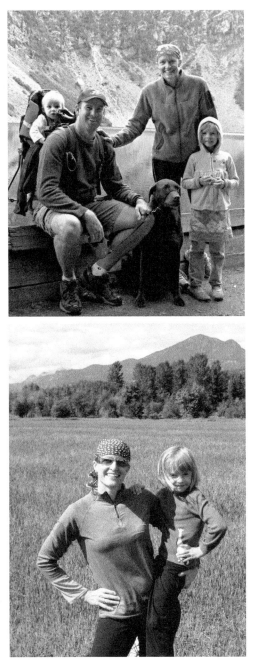

The Allison family goes hiking
in the North Cascades.

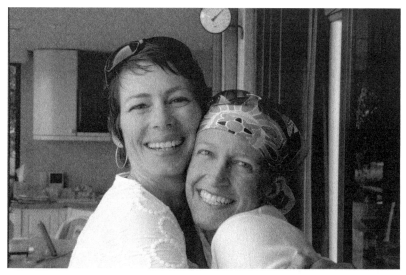

Visiting with Sharlyn, my "cancer guru".

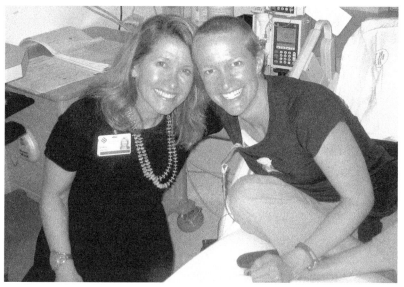

Visiting with Debora Jarvis towards the end of my treatments.

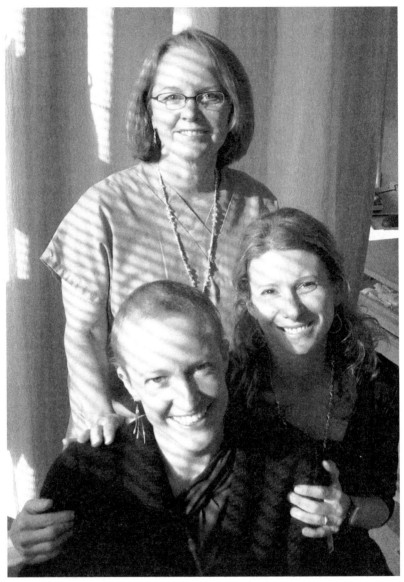

Nurses Sandy and Cathy with me on my last day of chemotherapy.

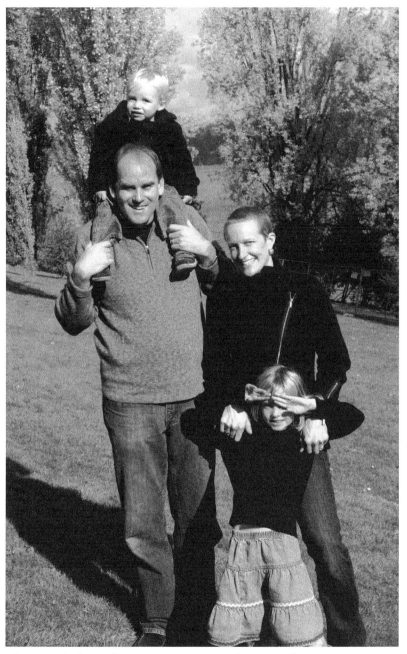

Done with chemotherapy, sporting a newly-sprouted crew cut; surgery and radiation still to go.

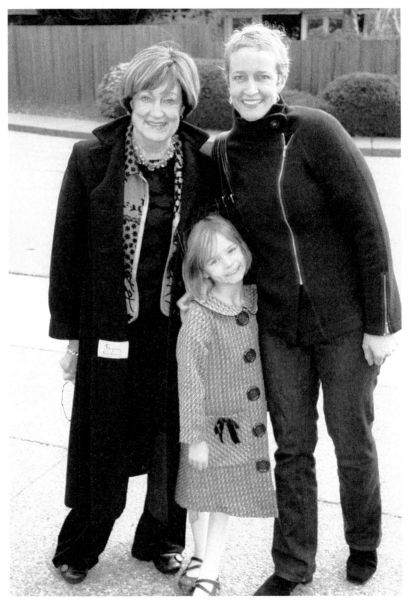

My mother, Maddy, and I (with a Labradoodle-like hairdo) at the end of radiation therapy.

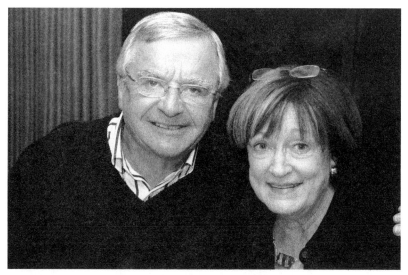

My fantastic parents, Bob and Emily.

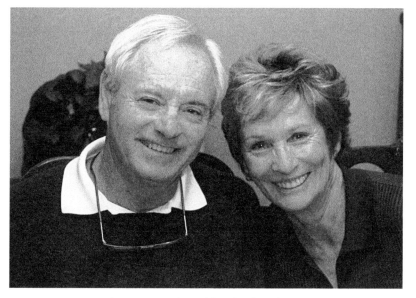

Ryan's mom, Gail, and her husband, Tommy.

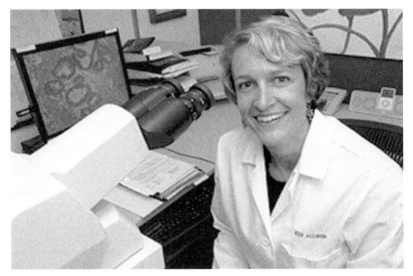

Back at work with my microscope.

Needles in My Forehead

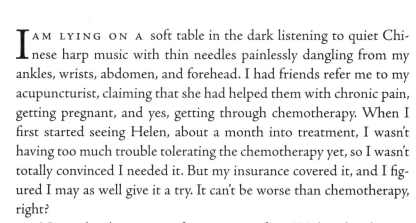

I AM LYING ON A soft table in the dark listening to quiet Chinese harp music with thin needles painlessly dangling from my ankles, wrists, abdomen, and forehead. I had friends refer me to my acupuncturist, claiming that she had helped them with chronic pain, getting pregnant, and yes, getting through chemotherapy. When I first started seeing Helen, about a month into treatment, I wasn't having too much trouble tolerating the chemotherapy yet, so I wasn't totally convinced I needed it. But my insurance covered it, and I figured I may as well give it a try. It can't be worse than chemotherapy, right?

Now it has become my favorite part of my Wednesday therapy routine. I am sure there are good things happening to my energy flow through the actual acupuncture, but the main reason I love it is even simpler: one complete hour of peace and quiet by myself. Powerful things can happen when you are in a room by yourself just trying to be still. You are left with nothing but your own thoughts for company and you get to know the depths of yourself quickly.

At first I try to make mental lists of the things I need to get done, replay recent events, or digest things that have been happening to me. But I have just finished reading Elizabeth Gilbert's *Eat, Pray, Love* and feel I should give meditation a shot. I believe strongly in the power of the mind to impact the physical body. I had learned firsthand already how mental fears can cause real physical symptoms and how the mind can be used to control them. I am no expert in meditation, but I know your mind can be incredibly powerful. And my acupuncture hour is the perfect opportunity to focus my mental energy on healing myself.

I refuse to be passive in my treatment. I may be passively receiving chemotherapy, radiation, even acupuncture, but I am actively choosing to believe in it working. And to succeed in something, you first have to believe what you are doing will make you succeed, no?

I take a deep breath and let myself sink into the table. My eyes are closed as I picture the thoughts in my mind clearing like clouds blown by the wind from a sunny sky. I try for mental silence. Quick blips of thoughts glow and fade on my mental screen like pegs in a Lite-Brite. I patiently dismiss them. I imagine my body filling with luminous, glowing energy. This I can feel physically as a slow surge that makes me feel both full and light. It is like I am on the edge of something fantastic, just about to leap in. It makes my fingertips and toes tingle. I am surprised to feel a rush just like that intoxication of a first love, running through me. What is this love I am feeling? It is an outpouring of love for myself and for my own physical being.

I love you! I find myself telling my own self over and over again.

You can do this, I tell my physical body. *You can conquer this. It is OK that you made a mistake, but you can help fix this now. I love you.* Tears are sliding down my cheeks as I lie there in absolute happiness.

And then I see her. She is familiar but older than me. Not my mother, not my grandmother, but *me.* I send myself a visit from my future self. She rests a hand on my shoulder gently and tells me everything will be all right. And I really feel like it will.

Sometimes I talk to the cancer or to the spirits in general. I say, *Can't you see how strong I am?!* And I picture myself glowing with energy. Or I envision my immune system circling and hunting down every last confused cancer cell in my body like a pack of hungry wolves, leaving me with nothing but a clean, healthy body. Whatever I focus on, I always walk out of my acupuncture sessions feeling more powerful than when I went in.

Dreaming of Barbie Boobs

I HAVE ARRANGED FOR A plastic surgery consultation to talk about breast reconstruction options. Ryan is also very obviously interested in this visit. This will be our first positive doctor's visit since we will actually be discussing life after cancer. What will my "reconstructed" self be?

I had been thinking more about whether or not to have bilateral mastectomies. My poor right side had really done nothing wrong. And there was no medical recommendation to prophylactically remove the unaffected side since I had tested negative for the known familial breast cancer gene mutations. I would be at a slightly increased risk of developing a second breast cancer because I had already had one, but modern imaging was getting so good I could just have frequent screening on the right side. And it certainly would not increase my survival from my current cancer.

No one was recommending this to me but myself. Part of it is because I have seen too much as a pathologist. I have seen the rare cases where a woman gets a second breast cancer in the opposite breast, or the rare cancers that were practically missed by all the fancy imaging. And I am not a woman who identifies particularly strongly with her breasts. I know that for some women the thought of losing one breast is heartbreaking, like losing a piece of herself. But oddly, I just don't feel all that strongly about them. I know I can be the same person without them, and frankly, I feel angry at them for betraying me. Plus, I did not want to always be compensating for asymmetries.

But more than anything, it feels empowering. I know it is extreme and it is definitely not for everyone, but I want them both gone.

Ryan and I sit in the examining room waiting for the plastic surgeon. I am wearing a gown and flashing him, making him laugh. We look through magazines for boobs we like as if they were catalogs we could show the surgeon. We are expecting him to come waltzing in carrying his samples of different silicone and saline implants. Or holding a big portfolio of his work we could browse through. But this is no Los Angeles nip-and-tuck clinic.

A medical student knocks and lets himself in. Ryan and I straighten up and get serious. The student runs through a series of questions with a level of confidence that surprises me. Was I ever this cool-headed with a patient? I am sure they always saw me sweat.

The plastic surgeon comes in. He has no photo album, no piles of sample implants to choose from. He frankly explains the reconstruction options to me. Post-mastectomy reconstruction typically involves either placing a saline or silicone implant or a tissue reconstruction "flap" from another area of the body to your breast. Because I am having post-mastectomy radiation I am not a candidate for immediate tissue reconstruction but I could do this after radiation is done. This surgery is complex and involves a lot of skill and surgical artistry. A section of abdominal fat is carefully removed so that the blood vessels feeding it stay intact and then it is reattached to vessels in the chest, creating a new breast that will wiggle and jiggle just like the real deal. But because it involves hooking up a new blood supply that if compromised would mean potential loss of the graft, you wake up in the ICU for monitoring. The recovery time is longer too. Not really easy fodder for the mother of a toddler and an infant.

The other option is to get implants. The surgeon explains differences between saline and silicone and how they place the implant beneath the pectoralis muscle. Usually, they first put in what is called a tissue expander at the time of surgery. The expander is basically an empty implant that can be accessed from your skin by a specific site to fill it up after surgery. It serves as a sort of place holder and is slowly filled with saline at serial visits so your tissue has a chance to slowly adjust to another size increase. You can keep getting them filled until they are the size you want and then you head back into surgery to get the expander exchanged for your permanent saline or silicone implants. Then, as the cherry on the sundae, you can get a tattoo of an areola and nipple reconstruction. I have joked with Ryan about how I would have the areola tattoo have a lacey edge or get his name etched in.

"Now let's take a look at you," the surgeon says with his charming accent.

I open my gown and show him what I've got.

"OK, so about an A to a light B cup with grade 1 ptosis." This means I have small, slightly droopy boobs.

"Hmmm. And let me see your abdomen . . . No, not enough extra tissue there to donate for a tissue reconstruction, I am afraid."

Is this a compliment? I don't have enough tummy fat to donate to my breasts?

"Well, let's see if you would have enough for donation of tissue from your rear area. Can you just wiggle those pants down a bit for me?"

I stand there awkwardly inching my pants down so that he can see how much of a "muffin-top" I have and turn my tail toward him. This is such an odd thing to be showing a colleague! *Look at my bum? Is it big enough?*

"Ah yes, ample tissue. We could do a flap from there after you are healed from radiation at some point."

Did he say "ample" tissue? Ryan is trying hard not to laugh. I guess how else can you put it? Yes, your butt is big enough to give up a little for some new boobs. What a victory. I knew having desert every night would pay off in some way, right?

"But if you don't want to wait for tissue reconstruction, given your breast size, I think we could place immediate implants at the time of surgery," he goes on.

"But I thought that I could not get any immediate reconstruction because I was going to have radiation?" I ask, confused. This was the one thing I thought was a given. No immediate reconstruction if you are even potentially getting post-mastectomy radiation, though I have to admit that I didn't really know why.

"Well, as long as your radiation oncologist is comfortable radiating an implant I think it can be fine. The chances of getting contracture on the radiated side are much higher; perhaps the majority of patients will get it. But the severity really varies and you can always go back to the OR and break up the capsule or exchange implants later. I have done this in a handful of patients who had post-mastectomy radiation."

This sounds like a good deal to me. I would not wake up flat-chested after surgery and have to go through all the adjustments to expand my chest slowly back to a reasonable size. I have a sudden urge to get out of there quickly before he changes his mind. And I am afraid my radiation oncologist will not like this idea.

"Well, I really like the idea of immediate implants," I tell him. "And I can always opt for tissue reconstruction later. Does this mean I can't really go any bigger?"

"Oh, you want to be bigger?" he asks, surprised.

"Uhhh. Well, I *am* pretty small now after having breast fed. Maybe back to my pre-baby B cup?" I ask hopefully. It *would* be nice to upgrade.

"I tell you what. I will put in the biggest size implant that will fit reasonably at the time of surgery," he compromises.

I picture him leaning over me in surgery urging on his team, "Get me the biggest one you've got. I think I can jam it in there. Come on, we can go bigger!" But he seems conservative and I somehow really doubt that I will wake up looking like Pamela Anderson.

I still feel like I haven't had a good image of what things will look like though.

"Do you have any photos? Nice examples?" I add.

"Oh yes. Let me go get the binder." And he disappears and quickly re-emerges with a thin white binder and begins flipping through it. There are laminated photos of women standing uncomfortably in very unflattering light. The ones with tissue reconstruction look like they had very recent surgery. Sutures are still in place and they look like they might have been victims of a very precise shark bite.

"These are the tissue reconstructions." He explains different aspects of where the scars are, etc. Once, one of my mother-in-law's friends came over to our house to talk with me about her experience with breast cancer. She took me into our bathroom and insisted on showing me her post-mastectomy tissue reconstruction. Locked in the bathroom, she lifted her shirt proudly to display two symmetrical, handsome bosoms. I would not have believed that one of those large fleshy breasts was not the real deal if it wasn't for one not having an areola tattoo yet. These photos were not doing this procedure justice. I guess there is nothing like seeing the real thing.

"These are the implant reconstructions." He goes on to the next page. "I call them Barbie Boobs." And he's right. They do look a heck of a lot like Barbie's nipple-less smooth mounds.

Well, sign me up for a pair like Barbie's got.

Finally I can feel like an all-American girl.

Good-Bye, Sunshine

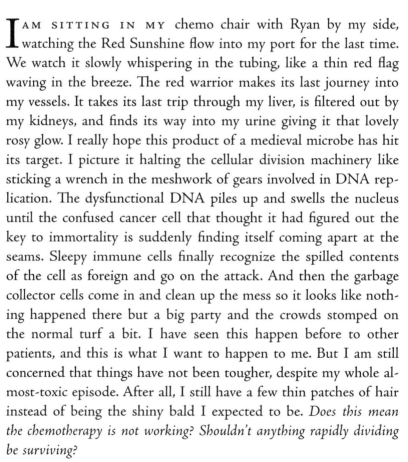

I AM SITTING IN MY chemo chair with Ryan by my side, watching the Red Sunshine flow into my port for the last time. We watch it slowly whispering in the tubing, like a thin red flag waving in the breeze. The red warrior makes its last journey into my vessels. It takes its last trip through my liver, is filtered out by my kidneys, and finds its way into my urine giving it that lovely rosy glow. I really hope this product of a medieval microbe has hit its target. I picture it halting the cellular division machinery like sticking a wrench in the meshwork of gears involved in DNA replication. The dysfunctional DNA piles up and swells the nucleus until the confused cancer cell that thought it had figured out the key to immortality is suddenly finding itself coming apart at the seams. Sleepy immune cells finally recognize the spilled contents of the cell as foreign and go on the attack. And then the garbage collector cells come in and clean up the mess so it looks like nothing happened there but a big party and the crowds stomped on the normal turf a bit. I have seen this happen before to other patients, and this is what I want to happen to me. But I am still concerned that things have not been tougher, despite my whole almost-toxic episode. After all, I still have a few thin patches of hair instead of being the shiny bald I expected to be. *Does this mean the chemotherapy is not working? Shouldn't anything rapidly dividing be surviving?*

I congratulate myself on having likely made it through the

worst of the chemotherapy. I can wean myself off the "G" shots and all the anti-side effect medication I was taking. It will be nice not to carry such a pharmacy with me everywhere and to not have to deal with needles and self-induced shots in the abdomen. But we leave the chemo suite behind unceremoniously since I will be back next week to start my new regimen. My next three months I will get Taxol (from the mighty Yew tree) and I will begin my year's worth of antibody therapy with Herceptin. I will start "chemo light."

The next week I am getting my mid-chemotherapy MRI to check on my progress. I am lying face down in that noisy machine. The loud bangs and beeps are not nearly drowned out by the soothing classical music they pipe into your headphones. I am hoping that the results will show the cancer melted away into darkness. I ask the radiologists if I can look at the MRI with them once they have read it, and they are nice enough to agree to take a break from their busy day to do so. Later that day, I am sitting in the dark reading room with them looking at my own images for the first time. They pull up my initial MRI from March to go over where we started from. There on the screen are my breasts in ghostly outline and the left one is very obviously filled with what looks like bumpy irregular clouds. All I can think is *my God, that is one of the biggest breast cancers I've seen.* And it's mine. It doesn't belong to a patient that I've never met and am presenting in conference but to *me*.

Next they pull up my current images. There they are again, my ghostly breasts, only this time they are much, much smaller since they are no longer lactating. And as they scroll through the images I am disappointed to see the storm clouds are still there. They are no longer one large thunderhead; they have broken off into smaller pieces, but they span the same 7 cm distance. So it is still there. There is less of it and it looks like it took a hit from the Red Sunshine, but a decent amount appears to be struggling for survival or is just undaunted by what we are attacking it with. *Damn.* I was hoping for some sort of miracle response. My radiology friend reminds me that I am only halfway through my treatment. That may be true, but weren't the biggest guns already unleashed? Aren't we following up with more friendly juice? I am suddenly missing the Red Sunshine.

But I remind myself that I will now be able to start on Herceptin—the fabulous new antibody therapy that has dramatically improved survival rates for HER2-positive cancers like mine when used with chemotherapy. And because it is targeted to the cancer only, it doesn't make you feel awful like chemotherapy does. I'm really lucky I will be able to take this drug, which was only approved for non-metastatic cancers like mine in the last couple of years. So there is just a different kind of sunshine to come.

The same week I also get another biopsy of the residual cancer because it is part of the research study I am enrolled in. I convince them to take a second biopsy for me to take back to our lab so I can take a look at it with my microscope. I want to see what exactly has the gall to still be around after all that toxic therapy. The next day I am holding the slide in my hands and am ready to face the beast again. Will it be mostly in situ carcinoma? I think, *hopefully*. In situ carcinoma is the kind that has not yet invaded, so it is less dangerous since it can't spread through the body. Often chemotherapy will wipe out the invasive cancer, but since it can't access the bad cells that have not broken through the normal duct structure as well, the in situ cancer can be all that is left behind. Maybe that is what my residual masses are. I lean my eyes up to the microscope and peer into the battle scene, and what I see makes my heart rate pick up. There is the same ugly invasive beast with its warped pink cell borders and malignant purple nuclei marching through the tissue like a team of army tanks. *Damn you!* I flip to a higher power and start talking smack to it again.

I will destroy *what is left of you, buddy*, I tell it. *You better pack your bags because the yew tree train and HER2 magic bullet are coming to town and you don't stand a chance.*

Then I go to another power higher and I begin to notice something strange. Most of the cancer cells are stuffed with neutrophils, which are usually only called in when there is an active infection.

But there they are inside the bubbly cytoplasm of the cancer cells. Are they eating them? Or being eaten? Am I basically looking at a graveyard of cancer cells? Are they victims on the battlefield being eaten by the vultures? They still look so life-like it is really tough to be sure if they are viable or not.

But maybe, just maybe, they are on their way out for good.

A Visit with My Cancer Guru

THE NEXT WEEKEND IS the Fourth of July holiday and we are headed down to visit my parents in the Bay Area. While we are there I am hoping to connect with my friend Sharlyn. She has been my guide through this whole endeavor. I call her with every question too personal for my doctors, and we compare notes on our decisions, emotions, and outcomes. She talked me through the shaky few days before my first dose of chemotherapy and sent me flowers on D-day. She has already passed through all the same doors I am now walking through.

I appreciate so much how willing she is to talk me through a process I am sure she would rather be putting completely behind her right now. Actually, because we originally met when she was dating a friend of ours a few years ago, I have not seen her in a long time. I remember her beautiful long dark hair and tall elegance. And since she moved from Seattle to San Francisco right after she was diagnosed we have only re-connected over the phone. I invite her over to my parents' house and am ecstatic that she has the time to stop by. My cancer guru is coming!

When the door bell rings I am surprised to see the same tall Sharlyn I remember but with short wavy dark hair in an overgrown pixie cut. That's right; she finished chemotherapy only six months ago, so her hair is not that long yet.

"Hi there, stranger!" I give her a hug and she leans back and looks at me.

"I like the scarf—nice look," she adds.

"I like the new boobs. Wow! You got a big new pair!" I notice the big round breasts peeking out the top of her low cut shirt and laugh at how I feel totally entitled to be staring at her chest.

"I know, I know. This shirt makes them look bigger though. Yeah, I like them!" She gives them a little clutch.

We go outside and sit on my parents' deck. My mom has put out cookies and coffee (love her!). Sharlyn turns down the sugar (the "cancer eats sugar" mantra) and we start talking about how she has changed her diet since her diagnosis.

Maddy pitter-patters around us while playing out some inner drama with a doll and a boat. We throw a ball in the water for Sharlyn's oversized Labrador and he enthusiastically entertains us as we catch up. We are two young women in our early thirties, sitting on a deck on a warm July day talking about getting our breasts removed, hair loss on chemotherapy and radiation skin changes. What could be better?

After we have covered a lot, she says "You know I sure felt angry about getting cancer. But you don't seem that angry, Kim."

This had not occurred to me before—to be angry about having cancer? I sure feel sorry for myself and still get scared, but anger had not been in my emotional spectrum yet. I see where she is coming from though. She had things taken away from her by cancer; she had to postpone her wedding day a year and has eggs harvested to hopefully someday be able to have kids. These are things I already have and I am suddenly incredibly grateful for. I would be pissed too if something put those opportunities at risk.

Why wasn't I angrier about this? Why was I so quick to accept it instead of rallying against the whole concept? Was it because I see how many women are diagnosed with breast cancer on a daily basis at work? It is not why me but why *not* me: it has happened to so many women whose names have crossed my microscope on their biopsy glass slides. I am the one who signs the report telling a woman for the first time that she has cancer. Why shouldn't it be me this time?

And it made me realize how different every person diagnosed with cancer reacts. It might make you angry. It might make you feel helpless or hopeless. It might make you feel more powerful. It might make you feel all of the above. There is no "right" way to deal with it—there is only *your* way to deal with it.

Good-Bye, Sunshine;
Hello, Yew Tree

M Y FIRST DOSE OF the mighty yew tree (Taxol) begins today. I finger my left breast absently on the car ride to the cancer center, feeling the soft but still lumpy area over the upper half. What if this tree bark therapy is too kind and gentle to get rid of any remaining cancer? Am I getting the most effective regimen for my cancer? How will we know it is working over the next three months?

I had asked my oncologist this question last time I saw her, and she had just answered, "Well, we won't since we won't get any imaging again until you are done."

So what if it *grows* on this therapy instead of further dissolving like it has over the last three months on Adriamycin and Cytoxan? My oncologist assures me this is extremely rare.

Hmmm, guess I will have to just have a little faith. We will know if it worked at the end if there is no cancer left when my breast leaves the surgeon's hands and is examined under a pathologist's microscope. If they don't see any residual cancer cells, then essentially it is like a cure (although never a total guarantee). If it doesn't all disappear, I will have to keep my fingers crossed that there wasn't any resistant cancer hiding somewhere else in my body that was not removed with surgery. And that would be a lot to hope for. In the trial I am enrolled in, I would get an extra three months of a different chemotherapy regime if there is residual cancer in the breast or lymph nodes removed at the time of surgery. But what I really, really want is a complete response to these six months of chemotherapy. This is what I am wishing for, focusing my energy on, and doing my magic for!

Taxol comes with its own unique set of possible side effects. There are still the usual pests of possible aches and pains, mouth sores, and the like, but Taxol can damage your nerve endings so that you get numbness and tingling in your feet or fingers, which is called peripheral neuropathy. Also, some people experience an initial allergic reaction to the first infusion.

My nurse preps me with all this information before I get my first dose.

"So because of the risk of allergic reaction, we'll give you a nice dose of antihistamines before you start getting your Taxol. You'll feel nice and sleepy. Then we will run the Taxol slowly over several hours and keep an eye on you as we infuse," she says.

"What would it look like if I had an allergic reaction?" I ask, envisioning me puffing up like a cherry tomato.

"Trouble breathing, flushing, or hives—but we can manage those if they happen and still give you the therapy." She knows I wouldn't want to be denied therapy from the way I reacted when I was temporarily denied my Red Sunshine. I need this juice to work!

"Oh goody. So, all this is going to take a while I guess," I answer.

In contrast to the Red Sunshine, which was over within half an hour, this chemotherapy will be more like what I was originally envisioning: long sessions hooked up to a big bag on a pole. Ryan and I settle in for the duration. This will be an extended version of our previous chemo-dates.

We start our date with the nice cocktail of IV Benadryl . . . mmmm a silly buzz drifts over me. The next course starts with me hardly noticing at all. What a cheap date I am. The nurse keeps checking on me to see if I am having any reactions. I keep waiting to suddenly feel my airways constrict and face flush with heat, but it never happens. The hours tick by. By seven o'clock at night I am ready for chemo-date desert, my first dose of the antibody therapy, Herceptin. By the end of it all, it is eight o'clock at night—a six-hour chemo-date record. I don't think I've ever had a date with Ryan that long before. And I must say the service was incredible.

Reunions

ONE OF THE AMAZING things about having something like cancer happen to you is that people from your past now want to reach out to you again. It can scare some people off, not because they aren't good friends but mainly because they don't know how to deal with it themselves. But really, there is no right or wrong way to let someone know you are thinking about them. I get a few hand-written letters from old friends letting me know they are thinking about me (one comes with a gift certificate for a manicure/pedicure). In this technology-savvy era I also get lots of electronic love in the form of text messages, e-mails, and comments on the CaringBridges blog I set up to keep everyone informed.

People want to know how you are doing and not bother you at the same time. So setting up this blog is the perfect way to both give me a therapeutic outlet for my experiences and to keep everyone up-to-date. It seems to spread like a virus through my past—finding even the least likely people. The older brother of a guy I used to carpool to school with, a girl I was on swim team with at age twelve, another that I haven't seen since I was probably eight years old, friends of friends, mom's of friends, people I have never even met but that have amazing words of encouragement for me. It is impossible to feel alone when you are getting site visits every time you write a new entry. And then there are some people who have been in your life before but now suddenly re-emerge as a prominent figure.

Naomi was like this. In high school we had a circle of six girlfriends: Joanna, Katie, Sheila, Abbi, myself, and Naomi. We stuck together against what seemed like the crazy adventure of freshman to senior year and then later stayed close enough that we were each bridesmaids in each other's weddings. We seemed to rotate who was closest with whom, but we were all part of the same gang. Naomi is the daughter of a rabbi and a social networking expert. She has always been big on loyalty and who meets her standards as a true friend. While this may have driven us crazy sometimes as we tried to navigate through the complex social system of high school, as we got older her high standards of friendship made it clear that she was someone you could really lean on when you needed her. I remember being so thankful she was one of my bridesmaids when I got married because she was the only one actually concerned with how everything was going to go rather than being totally distracted by hair, dresses, and chitchat. And now, suddenly it feels great to have her checking in on me with phone calls every week asking how I am doing. She has grown up and become a good Jewish mother. She even calls *my* mother asking her what she can do to help her, giving her recipes to try next time she comes up to visit me. She researched books on cancer for kids and even sent us a "chemo doll" (named "Kim" of all things!) that came complete with all three hair stages; long hair that was removable for the chemo bald look and then a short mossy-looking hair cap to show what it would look like when it first re-sprouted. Maddy, of course, was curious about that doll, but it quickly lost favor against her more "beautiful" Barbie dolls that still had long gorgeous hair and big boobs.

Abbi was my oldest friend. She and I were best buddies back in third grade, when we imagined ourselves the queens of mischief. We would skip out on our summer sailing class if it looked too windy for our tiny El Toros (which were basically the size of bathtubs and no match for the winds of the San Francisco Bay) and hide out. Once, we even "borrowed" enough change from the dashes of a few convertibles in the parking lot to pay for a fare on the Angel Island ferry instead of rigging our little boats for a sailing race. We shipped ourselves off to the island only to discover that her little brother's camp was also on the island that day. We spent the afternoon hiding out in bushes, behind picnic tables and trees, feeling like spies and fugitives. Later, we fed the not-so-wild raccoons crackers that were placed between our toes from delicately outstretched legs.

That was probably the craziest thing we both ever did as kids. And we did it together. We were inseparable from third to sixth grade, and then I moved back east for three years until we were reconnected in high school when I moved back. In high school we had similarly innocent adventures but this time sneaking around high school parties as a freshman, terrified of both the people and the activities, and would rush back to one of our houses for a nice safe slumber party complete with Entenmanns's fat-free snack food and popcorn. There was something enchanting about Abbi that made you want to be around her and giggle with her and be just like her. Tall and super thin (from both a superfast metabolism and a finicky diet) with long thick blond hair and a flat chest, she was a beautiful late bloomer. She had hardly even kissed a boy in high school, fell in love in college, and ended up marrying the boy she lost her virginity to. She later went on to get a PhD in child psychology. Now she lives in New York City with her husband and their two little boys.

Then there was Sheila. She was six feet tall and awkward in high school. We spent many a weekend together making mix tapes and dreaming about boys we would never date. I would spend summers with her at her family's cabin in Lake Tahoe and we would walk to the beach and look for people to play volleyball with, suntan, and listen to more mix tapes. Her best mix was one that featured Vanilla Ice, Easy-E, and Millie Vanilli. And since "Ice Ice Baby" was one of her favorite songs, it was on there twice in a row for extra listening pleasure. We felt like hip suburban white girls in our clean-cut world rapping about "bitches and hoes."

She was incredibly self-conscious of her height the first few years of high school. So much so that she once pulled down her kneepads in the middle of a volleyball game when she noticed a guy she had a crush on walk in the gym (she thought they made her legs look like stilts). By the summer of our senior year, we had finally grown into our looks enough, shed our braces, and emerged as college-ready babes. And by then Sheila's height made her look like a supermodel. But the funny thing was she was also legally blind without her two-inch-thick glasses, which of course she was too embarrassed to wear in social situations. So I often had to pre-screen any innocent tall guy for their cuteness level for her. I was the ultimate nonthreatening "wing woman." We visited each other many times during college since we both went back east for our higher learning, and every time we saw each other it was like time had never passed. Crazy to think that now she is pregnant with her second child (this is the same woman who once told me when I was pregnant with Maddy "Pregnancy seems creepy because you are never really alone . . .") and living back in Marin working as a child psychologist.

Katie was the bubbly one who could fill a room with her giant smile and bedroom eyes. The oldest girl in a family of six, she had a nurturing way about her from helping take care of her younger siblings (we voted her most likely to have kids first in our group—although somehow I managed to claim that title in the end.) She was the only one of us under five foot seven (and only by a few inches I think) and she was also the only one who was actually what you could describe as well-endowed. This definitely drew more attention from the boys in high school, and she was envied by the rest of us for having an actual serious boyfriend at the time. But she was the center of a huge high school controversy when that very same boyfriend decided to take up with another friend of ours at the same time. In the end, the dramatic break-up brought her closer to us, and we had much more fun prowling around together than when she was off with her old boyfriend and his friends. She went on to UC Santa Barbara, got her teaching degree, and is now a kindergarten teacher and mother of two, living in Los Angeles.

Joanna was the studious athlete and confidant. Tall and muscular, she was a star of the volleyball, basketball, and soccer teams. She was also student body president and drove a Volvo. She was the cornerstone of many freshman-year slumber parties, and she had an amazing way of making you feel like you were her most important friend in the whole world. We were kindred spirits in a lot of ways. We were both focused on academics and very goal-oriented but liked the idea of a balanced lifestyle. Both of us ended up applying to Princeton, getting in, and becoming even closer in our four years there. She switched sports to rowing, and it was through her that I discovered how fantastic the rower-boys were (and really how I met Ryan). My third and fourth years of medical school I lived with her in New York City, where she was enduring the work hard, play hard lifestyle of a job in finance and I was pretty much working hard and studying hard. She was there to convince me to stay in medical school when I would come home exhausted, jaded, and convinced I needed to move to Seattle immediately to join Ryan. We managed to lead parallel lives from our teenage years to our mid twenties, when I moved to Seattle and she moved across the ocean to London. It was there that she met a handsome Brit, got married, quit the intensity of her finance career, and is now trying to get pregnant, playing tennis, and taking cooking classes (sounds good to me!).

So the girls have been planning a reunion. Cancer inspires these. Sheila can't come because she is too pregnant and Abbi has just moved to New York City and has her hands full. But Joanna is flying all the way from London, Katie from Los Angeles, and Naomi from the Bay Area. I can't wait to see my girls! It feels as though time has never passed when you get together with such good friends from your past.

And here they are—a pregnant Katie, newlywed Joanna, and mother–of-two Naomi, all grown up and complete women. But we of course still see only the high schoolers hidden beneath the thirty-something exteriors. We start talking and we don't stop the entire weekend.

The first night we are at Ryan's restaurant on Mercer Island (Cellar 46), enjoying a bit of wine on the deck and catching up. Naomi suddenly turns the conversation focus on me and how I am dealing with my "situation." They ask me all kinds of questions. Naomi even throws out "Do you still have *sex?*" Which I realize is a legitimate question and makes me laugh. (And yes we do, thank you very much.)

I tell them how one of the hardest things is watching my kids and knowing that I might not be there for them in a few years.

"You know your kids will be OK, right, Kim?" Naomi tells me.

And somehow this sets off a wave of emotion so strong I can't hold it back. To hear that out loud for the first time for some reason just makes me lose it. I am crying my eyes out and several of them start to as well. The waiter comes by to tell us about the wines and quickly turns on his heels as he sees the table of whimpering women.

I know my kids will be OK without me. At the same time, I don't want anyone to be OK without me. And I don't want anyone else to acknowledge that I might not be around to raise them.

Once we all get a hold of ourselves we manage to move on to lighter topics. But it feels good to have let loose with old friends. We spend the rest of the night gossiping about wayward antics in high school, updating each other on other people from our past, and talking about who has "Facebooked" who. Wow. We are in high school again. Naomi and Katie actually convince me to join in the Facebook trend, which apparently isn't just for teenagers anymore.

Later that weekend we all go to cheer on my brother in his first sprint triathlon. Since I wouldn't let him shave his head in my honor, he refocused his empathetic energy on doing this race for me. He even pulled off the drama of crossing the finish line and then placing his participation metal around my neck. Aw . . . shucks, little brother.

At the end of the weekend, I am sad to see the gang fade away back to their husbands and kids. Seeing old friends is a lot like visiting your old self, really. It was fun to travel back in time to revisit who we were almost twenty years ago, realize how much we have grown and also how much the core of who we are and who we were is the same.

On the Hot Flash

THE DREADED HOT FLASH that menopausal memoirs are written about finally starts taking hold of me. Strangely enough I actually think I like them. They are like an angry force being unleashed. And it is so fascinating to me that the shutdown of my ovaries can cause this irregular outburst of thermal energy—like they are pissed off about being forced into retirement and are letting the rest of the body know their last bits of power.

The heat starts in my feet and steadily travels up my legs. It warms up my core and then comes my favorite part: it blasts through my rooftop. I can feel my head releasing heat and I picture steam rising off my bald head. It feels like this release must be visible. I am a steamy bald-top—a volcano of end-stage ovarian energy. The force of it makes me feel powerful. Forget quiet little old lady—menopause is like a lion roaring.

Clearly the novelty wears off after a while, especially when I have to wake up in the middle of the night and throw off my covers to keep from being boiled alive, only to be freezing five minutes later as the sweat dries on my skin. But I try to not be too dramatic about them when they hit. I lean into them and let the warm tide pass over me until it has left again. This too will pass . . .

Turning a Corner

SOMEHOW AROUND MONTH FOUR I feel like I turn a mental corner. I stop fixating on my death and start seeing my future. I stop spending hours on the Internet searching for articles that may show better outcomes than the fairly grim ones I have read. I stop picturing my children's lives without me. At least, I don't do it *constantly*.

It is like I had to imagine the whole set of worst case scenarios, come to terms with them, and digest them like a huge bolus of greasy food and then let them go. The constant lump in my throat is gone. The feeling that I am pretending when I tell people I am going to be fine is gone. I am beginning to really believe it now. I can't explain what it is that made the change. It was a slow dissolving of a fog of doubt and fear and suddenly I am standing happily in the sunshine again. I know that life has no guarantees and I am becoming OK with that. If the damn thing comes back, then it comes back and if I die young, well, ain't that glamorous! But I am not so afraid of my future anymore.

I decide to start looking and planning for the long term as much as possible. I go back to work on Thursdays and work on projects that have a long timeline to completion. I play with my kids without letting my mind wander to when they might miss me and instead turn to what I can be teaching them now.

I see my great-aunt Elsmarie a few times during the course of my treatment. She was diagnosed with stage four ovarian cancer about six months before my diagnosis. She is fighting a very tough diagnosis with strength. I have seen how raw her fear is and how it grips her into a state of panic every time her tumor marker tests are checked. I know the feeling. This isn't the journey we signed up for. I still struggle with the crushing weight that fear can bring down on me. But now I am at least beginning to understand that it is a sense of peace that I most wish for anyone facing their mortality or dealing with a serious life crisis. Giving up your fear does not mean you are giving in, it just gives you more strength to face the road ahead. Easier said than done, I know.

Shaman

I HAVE BEEN CONTEMPLATING SEEING a naturopath just to explore what this complementary medicine may have to offer. I have been taking all my conventional therapy, but I still have an urge to make sure there isn't something else out there I should be looking into. I make an appointment with one of the naturopaths that my nutritionist recommended. She was originally trained as a nurse and was considered well-versed in what could potentially interact with my chemotherapy and other drugs, and I consider this extremely important. So I show up and quickly learn that seeing a naturopath is really not that different from going to a good traditional doctor. You get asked lots of questions about your medical history and are also asked how you are doing emotionally. But in the end what they recommend is drugs. They are natural compounds but they are certainly not consumed in any more natural of a way than conventional drugs. And while I realize that adding things like extra vitamin D to my diet may be a good idea, I really don't want to be adding another batch of expensive pills to my already full medicine cabinet.

I leave feeling unsatisfied with how clinical the whole experience was. I think what I was really looking for was an old-fashioned "medicine woman." Someone with deep wrinkles and eyes linked to the spirits who could lay their hands on me and feel the evil leave as they cast their energy against it—an old-fashioned healer. Despite my obvious faith in conventional medicine, I find the idea of a magical healer both fascinating and appealing. But these people probably only exist in the darkest depths of tribal forests.

I write about my disappointment in my cancer blog that night and half-jokingly ask if anyone knows a good shaman. I am surprised the next day to receive e-mails from a few people recommending an actual practicing shaman. One woman tells me she used to work at AT&T with a woman who was also a shaman. *Hmmm. Not exactly my vision of the ancient medicine woman I had in my head—she can hook you up with a great phone plan* and *perform miracles . . .* I decide to look online for more information on these modern oracles. I Google "Seattle Shaman" and get a funny array of Web sites featuring predominantly white women who look like they are playing dress-up, clad with Native-American accents over brightly patterned clothes from Ross Dress for Less. Forget it. I realize that the wise ancient Native-American miracle worker most likely doesn't have a Web site, much less a computer, and I let it go.

The next week I am dropping my daughter off at preschool when I run into another student's father, who was recently diagnosed with a low-grade lymphoma.

"How are you doing?" I ask him.

"Great, I am actually seeing a shaman," he replies abruptly.

What?! OK, a shaman had officially found me. I have to explore this further. Three weeks later I am knocking on the door of her house. A thin woman with long grey hair answers and ushers me inside. Her house is neatly arranged with small spiritual knick-knacks carefully placed on book shelves. It smells like freshly burnt sage. I sit on a little couch as she asks me a few questions about my history. She is friendly and smiling. She is also a cancer survivor. We connect over our idle talk, and I wonder if she chats with the spirits in the same easy way.

When we are done talking, she makes a little bed of blankets for me on the floor and gives me an eye pillow. She tells me to relax and then calls out to the spirits to join us. Then she gets quiet and starts to shake a rattle. She shakes and shakes and shakes that rattle—for probably thirty minutes at least. I try to meditate. I focus on feeling the energy of the visiting spirits, but I think, *I should not have had that single tall latte this morning because my mind will not sit still.* I do feel some energy surging through me every once in a while and try to imagine that there are spirits all around me. Then I figure my shaman is the one who really needs to make contact so I go ahead and unleash my mind to run wherever it pleases. I run through to-do lists and think of places I want to travel to, and then try to focus on the spirits again. *Be still, grasshopper, be still.* It is clearly time for some guided meditation CDs.

When the rattle finally stops shaking, she starts telling me what she learned. She blows the healing energy and lost pieces of my soul she has recovered back into my heart and the top of my head. What did she tell me? I guess I have to say visiting the spirit world is like going to Vegas—and what happens in Vegas stays in Vegas. But I will reveal that my spirit animals are the wolf and the butterfly *(who knew you could have two?).* She did not magically prophesize too much on my future, although she did tell me I am on the right career path and that she saw my long-term future. She emphasized that I should try and keep balance in my life and visualize positive outcomes. It is a bit like seeing a therapist, but there are extra psychic powers mixed in with your therapy session.

She also mentions retrieving a lost piece of my soul from a traumatic experience when I was seventeen years old that made me lose my sense of security about the world around me. At first I thought her timing was a few years off—I had lost a close friend in a car accident in high school, but I remembered it as my freshman year. Later, as I thought more about it, I remembered that my friend's parents had just found out she had gotten into her top choice college so it must have been junior year . . . when I was seventeen. The spirits were right after all.

At the end she hands me a CD recording of all that she said, along with a small agate. It feels strange to pay at the end of this immaterial experience, and I can't help but think about what a nice little business she has—working from home, making a few hundred dollars a session. She even has a personal assistant. Maybe I should consider a career change—but alas, my mind could never be so still.

All in all, I am happy I have explored this avenue. She did give me a feeling of comfort and confidence in the future, and I like the feeling of angels and spirits watching over me despite my atheism. I am still convinced my own mind is one of the most powerful tools I have in my recovery. And if visualizing a positive outcome doesn't actually ensure one, at least it makes it a more positive experience.

Looking My Age

I HAD ANOTHER DOSE TODAY and then ran off to Maddy's preschool beginning-of-the-year BBQ. It is a windy but sunny evening and the kids are happily running around from the park beach to our picnic tables strewn with potluck goodies. I remember being at the first of these "meet the other parents" gigs. I think I was as shy as my two-and-half- year-old daughter. All the other parents seemed to know each other from the year before and I assumed that I was the only "awful" working mom. But I quickly learned that many of the moms worked too (with a fair number of stay-at-home dads) and after two years I felt like I had made friends with many of the parents.

I am not sure what all the new moms think of the mom in the headscarf. I should have worn a name tag stating, "Maddy's mom, currently fighting cancer"—it would have been a nice conversation starter. I think I may lose the headscarf soon anyway—I actually went to work a few times without it now that I have a fuzzy covering of hair like a baby bald eagle.

Maybe they thought I had to cover my hair for religious reasons. Or maybe they just thought I was a really old mom wearing some sort of old-fashioned scarf hairdo—like I had curlers under it or something.

Actually, the last time I went in for a check-up with my oncologist the nurse who was taking my vitals saw in my chart that my birthday was approaching and asked me if I would be celebrating "the big 5-0."

The big 5-0?

The big 5-0!

I slowly digested this and laughed it off.

"No, try my thirty-fourth birthday—thank you!"

Come on now. I am a glamorous vision of a young chemo patient. She must have been used to the older patient demographic in the clinic. But I guess my hair *is* coming in an ashy color that *is* hard to tell if it has blonde or grey mixed in. *But it is dirty* blonde, *damn it!* I *do* have darker circles and a more puffy appearance under my eyes. My eyebrows are still really light and my eyelashes are only tiny stumps, which make me look washed out. Maybe I do look fifty. Or close to forty at least. And I *am* in menopause.

At least my boobs will always be perky. Someday I will be fifty and graying, but my boobs will still look like a teenager's, minus a few scars.

So there.

Dragonfly Nymphs

THIS MORNING I GO with Maddy's school on a field trip
to investigate ponds in Discovery Park. The teacher, Miss Su-
san, and a few other moms slowly herd the curious pack of a dozen
four-year-olds through the woods to a series of ponds. Ranger Jim,
who looks like Jiminy Cricket with his long grasshopper-like face,
leads the way with tales of frog eggs and dragonfly nymphs. Because
it has not rained in so long the ponds are covered with a thin film
of tiny bugs, plants and debris—like a layer of dirty, silvery icing.
The kids use fishnets to scoop up whatever creatures are lurking in
the murky water and come screaming when they find anything that
wiggles. We find tiny fish, dragonfly nymphs (who knew dragonflies
spent their pre-flight days underwater as a spastic worm-like bug?),
water skimmers, backswimmers, and even a tiny leech. My favorite
is the backswimmer, a legume-sized creature that rows himself
around upside down with two large oar-like hind legs. I am getting
muddy and dipping my hands in pond water. I get excited when a
tadpole is finally found. Did I ever picture myself doing this while
on chemotherapy?

After a quick picnic lunch I drop Maddy at home with our
au pair, Halia, and I am off to the cancer center for my afternoon
chemotherapy cocktail. I am reminded of work again as soon as I
am near the building and the let-down from my field-trip buzz hits.
Work seems unusually busy right now with abstracts for meetings
due, conferences to give, and the ever-increasing numbers of breast

cancer cases to review. After several months of my new reality, where I was feeling like work was a good distraction, I am starting to feel like I am reaching a new tipping point of busyness. I am waking up at night thinking about work, instead of worrying about cancer or my kids. It is starting to feel like I am keeping myself only inches above a rising flood of activity. Even on my day off I am rushing around to a bunch of appointments all day. And I am not sure I like it.

As I sit in my chemotherapy chair editing a paper, bags of deliciousness dripping into my port, my favorite chaplain peeks her head around my privacy curtain.

"Oh my God," she says dramatically. She looks like she has tears in her eyes.

"Oh my God, I just resigned." She bursts out as she enters my room while wiping her hands with sanitizer lotion.

"What? Are you kidding me?" I answer back in shock. Here is a woman who clearly loves the work she does and she is resigning? What is going on?

"Well, I have been traveling a ton to give talks and then rushing back to work and seeing my patients. And I think it is just getting to be too much." She has been traveling the country giving talks about death and dying and her book—but of course with her trademark sense of humor that makes her wisdom go down easier.

"So you just decided to stop seeing patients?" I ask, curious as to how she came to her seemingly abrupt decision.

"Well, no. I have been thinking about it for a few months. And it has been causing me a ton of anxiety. I mean, not seeing patients?! I love my job, right? Then the other day I woke up and decided to try on the decision of not seeing patients right now—and it was like a weight had been lifted. So I knew it was time to leave." As she says this, she is getting tearful. This was clearly not an easy decision. But I find myself feeling a tinge of jealousy for her. She is at the end of something but about to start a new chapter in her life. And I would not be surprised if I saw this dynamo on *Oprah* someday soon.

I miss the feeling of a million new doors opening. That feeling has crystallized in my memory to a single moment when I was eighteen years old. I was sitting outside after dark shortly before heading off to college looking up at the night sky and there was this vast, endless universe sparkling down at me. I remember feeling like the world was mine to be discovered and no possibility was off-limits. I could take as many different paths as there were stars in the sky that night. My future was so undecided. That feeling lasted through much of college as I explored and learned with hunger. Even in medical school I loved discovering the workings of our internal solar systems and trying on different specialties. But then eventually as you move forward, doors close behind you. You get on a track and you ride it and suddenly it would be very complicated to get back off. Don't get me wrong, I don't regret the decisions I have made and I really like where I have ended up. But that moment where there is a break and a chance to change directions is enticing.

"What will you do next?" I ask, waiting to hear about all her fantastic ideas for her next endeavors.

"Rest, be present," she says.

Be present—and what of all the possible plans? What about the shiny future? Ah yes, grasshopper, don't forget the art of being still. Look for dragonfly nymphs and backswimmers in a pond on a sunny day. Or sit in a quiet spot and close your eyes and just breathe—without thinking of all the things you have to do or the things you wish you had time for. Daydream and you will feel the doors reopen. Plus, isn't that when you can hear yourself best?

One more dose to go!

Is It Gone but Not Forgotten?

I FINISH MY LAST TAXOL infusion uneventfully. I say good-bye to my nurses until at least after surgery in October, when I will be back every three weeks to complete my year's worth of Herceptin antibody therapy. I have managed to avoid the dreaded peripheral neuropathy (I have been taking tons of this odd-tasting glutamine powder to ward it off) and have also managed to gain back all the weight I had lost on Red Sunshine plus a little extra for good measure (amazing how fast your metabolism slows down in menopause). My hair has even started to grow back. It really did seem a kinder, gentler regime.

But was it working on the cancer? I had an end-of-therapy MRI to answer that very question and was waiting patiently at work for the results. I was disappointed by my mid-therapy MRI and was preparing myself for the worst possibility: no progress.

I knew there was no fairness in this game of life. I had seen active heroin addicts have complete responses to therapy and young mothers die of their disease. Even if my MRI did show residual disease, it was really only the pathology at the end of it all that would have the best answer. Sometimes only the in situ carcinoma, that can't spread beyond the breast, is left behind and shows up on imaging but the life-threatening invasive carcinoma is completely eradicated. So as all pathologists know, no matter what the imaging shows, it is "the *tissue* that is the issue." Still, it sure would be comforting to at least have a great response on imaging.

I try to distract myself at work all day, waiting for the call from the radiology department. Finally, the phone rings and the head of the breast imaging department is on the line.

"Hi Kim. I am looking at your MRI here," she says in a friendly and familiar voice.

"Yes? How does it look?" I am perfectly still. The clock on the wall has stopped and everything in the room is suddenly suspended in time.

"Kim, it's gone. It's completely gone. I see background changes here, but I think you have had a complete imaging response to therapy." She says these blessed words and time begins again, the clock ticks, my heart beats again and everything falls back into place. Order is restored.

"You're kidding me. Oh my god, you're kidding me." I want to drop the phone right then and start screaming and running down the hallways telling everyone I can find.

"Thank you, thank you, thank you! That is the best news I have heard in a long time!" I continue to thank her, hang up the phone, and *then* run up and down the halls telling everyone I can find.

I still am cautiously optimistic. I know that cases with complete imaging responses can still have scattered bits of invasive cancer that can't be seen because they no longer make a mass. I know this is not necessarily the answer to my atheist prayers.

But it is still damn good news.

Pre-Surgery Jitters

OH CRAP, I'M HAVING my boobs cut off. The reality of it is settling in rather unsettlingly. I have a date set—October 8. I am only taking a few weeks between finishing chemotherapy and having surgery. I want to get it over with. I am obsessive about planning everything. The kids will be sent down to my parents in California for a week so I can recover without having them trying to climb all over me. I am not even going to be able to pick up Henry for several weeks after surgery. What am I going to do, throw a rope down to him so he can climb out of his crib after a nap if I am home alone with him? *I'll figure it out, I am sure.*

The real problem is I that am just starting to feel relatively normal again. I am getting used to the routine of chemotherapy. I know I can handle it and go about my business as usual. And now the reality of knowing I am going in for surgery is making me sit up and remember—*fuck, I have cancer!*

October is breast cancer awareness month and everything has turned pink. The grocery store is stocked with pink items adorned with the breast cancer awareness ribbons. I receive three big bags of pink M&Ms from various friends. The newscasters are wearing pink on Channel 5. Target practically has a whole pink aisle. Even the NFL has decorated football players with pink ribbons on their helmets. It looks so odd to have those delicate ribbons on such husky men.

Everything seems decked out for the occasion of my breasts going away. Should I throw them a going away party?

Too morbid?

I cannot believe these things cross my mind.

Of course October is also Halloween so the orange and black
are out as well. Our house is on a busy street, so we have had a grand
total of zero trick-or-treaters in the last five years. Thus, I usually
don't decorate the yard too much. But this year I have a five-year-
old who has graduated from everything princess to everything
Scooby Doo and is very interested in all things spooky. So we hit the
drugstore and check out the selection of low-end Halloween décor.
Maddy is fascinated by the skeletons, mummies, and bloody body
parts available for purchase. She decides we need some gravestones,
spiders, a ghost, and a skeleton for the yard. I consider her requests.
Are gravestones too tacky for a house where a cancer patient lives? I
decide it is probably a faux pas only I would get, so I end up adding
them to the tab. When we get home, I put the tombstones beneath
a tree in our front yard. Then I put two small pumpkins at the base
of each of them, right under the RIP. I think they look like bright
orange breasts. This is the RIP shrine to my breasts. They will be
gone soon, floating peacefully in a Tupperware full of formaldehyde.
I shudder. May they rest in peace.

The Surgery

THE DAY OF SURGERY approaches faster than I anticipated. We send the kids off with my parents for a week of fun in California while I will convalesce. Suddenly the day is here. It is early in the morning the day of the surgery and I am pissed I can't have a latte or any breakfast. I have done all my positive visualization exercises to help with rapid healing and right now am just trying to distract myself and Ryan from the reality of what is about to occur.

Before surgery I get changed into one of those dreary hospital gowns. I'm then sent over to the nuclear medicine department to have some radioactive dye injected in my right breast so the surgeons can locate my sentinel lymph node in the OR. It is about 8:00 AM and I run into a few surgeons that I know on the way and wave to them. They look a bit confused and wave back. They are probably wondering how they know this patient and not recognizing it is their friendly pathologist colleague. Another colleague does my sentinel node studies with a handsome young resident who painlessly injects the radioactive material beneath my nipple. I walk around a bit waiting for the radioactivity to drain from my breast to the first draining ("sentinel") lymph node. I then get positioned beneath a large dinosaur of a machine that visualizes the radioactivity emitted. I get an "X" marking a spot in my armpit to help the surgeons find the magical node and I'm sent back to the pre-operative area.

Ryan and I do crosswords to stay busy, which we have never attempted together before, and we discover we are actually pretty good as a team. We meet my anesthesiologist, chat more, and sign consent forms for both the breast surgeon and the plastic surgeon. The pre-OP zone is a calm quiet area with the patients all corralled into bays with curtains for privacy. Heated blankets keep us warm and nurses keep us company. Staff in scrubs float by, peeking into bays, looking for their patients. There is not the moaning and groaning of the post-OP areas. It reminds me of the triage area in the Labor and Delivery ward, where I was only fourteen months ago about to give birth to Henry. Only it is strangely calmer than the tumultuous rollercoaster of giving birth. All the moves of this hospital visit are pre-planned, unlike the uncertainties during delivery. I think that in a lot of ways this is actually easier than giving birth. I just sit back, relax and let the surgeons do all the work. No one will be telling me to push or breathe. I won't have to ask for an epidural, they'll have me totally under so I won't feel a thing. But I guess I shouldn't really compare the two until after the surgery is over. And I can't exactly say that I would rather be having bilateral mastectomies than giving birth right now (although the thought of a third baby at this point does make me kind of queasy).

The time to be wheeled into surgery finally arrives and as my gurney rolls through the OR double doors, I am blowing kisses to Ryan, who smiles and waves. *This is going to be fine,* I tell myself. *I am going to be fine. This is not the last time I will see him. I am going to be fine.* Then the Versed kicks in and I am off to la-la-land.

Pain Cave

I WAKE UP AND AM initially confused about whether the surgery has taken place. Then I feel soreness in my throat and I can feel the place that the intubation tube was pressing against my upper lip. Yes, my surgery is over and I am in the recovery area. My vision is still blurry despite having my glasses on but I can tell that my chest is wrapped tightly in bandages and a Velcro bra of sorts. There is a feeling of great pressure across my chest. Ryan is next to me along with a nurse. They ask me how I am feeling and I try to speak but find my voice has gone incredibly hoarse from the intubation. They try to move my gurney and I feel a huge wave of nausea, which makes them quickly re-park me and push some anti-nausea cocktail through my IV and stick a scopolamine patch behind my ear. The anesthesiologist had warned me about this before surgery. But it is quickly gone and I just lie there trying to focus my blurry vision and trying to stay awake. My surgeons stop by to tell me that they felt the surgery was a success and I had only mild blood loss. Ryan wants to talk but I can barely keep my eyes open. We wait and wait for someone to transport us to the floor where I will spend my first night in the hospital since medical school (besides the Labor and Delivery ward).

Eventually I get sent upstairs and settled into a nice private room. It is around 7 PM. It was a six-hour surgery including the bilateral mastectomies, axillary dissection, sentinel lymph node, and reconstruction with implants.

My nurse cheerfully introduces herself. I try to give an upbeat quip to identify with her, but I am too out of it to come up with anything but hoarse answers to her questions. Ryan tries to joke with me a bit, but I still just want to go back to sleep mid-conversation. Plus laughing hurts my chest.

I spend the night trying not to move and falling in and out of sleep between rounds of vital signs. They take my blood pressure on my leg since I have an IV in my right arm and had my axillary dissection on the left. There are big signs in my room that say "No BP in arms" but it looks like "No BP in anus" because of the handwriting. One of the nurses notices this too and laughs as he changes it. I picture a large blood pressure cuff wrapped around my rear end—*no, thanks.*

I still have a catheter in, so I don't even need to get out of the bed to go to the bathroom. My urine is a strange toilet-bowl-cleaner green-blue from the sentinel lymph node dye used in surgery. I have three grenade-sized drains handing off long thin tubing that disappears into my Velcro bra and apparently is in my wound site to keep fluid from collecting. The nursing staff periodically empties red fluid from the drains as I lie half-asleep.

I am in a strange state of painful stillness.

Before 7:00 the next morning a herd of medical students and residents march into the room to wake me up and check on me. This used to be me! *How strange to be the one on the other side now, lying in the bed looking groggy and immobile.* They look excited to see me. They know I am a doctor here and want to chat. But I feel like my chest was just run over by a truck. I ask them if there was one in the OR yesterday and they laugh. I feel pretty awful. They are telling me about how I am going to get out of bed today, walk around, eat and drink, etc. And it sounds to me like they are asking for the moon. They tell me I look great but I don't believe them for a minute. My eyelids are still greasy from the ointment they put on in the OR before taping them closed so they don't dry out. And I am just getting enough hair back to look like I have bedhead with tufts sticking out straight on both sides.

The plastics team whizzes in as well and seems to push back the surgery team as they undo the Velcro on my fancy bra to check my incisions. I try to see what they are looking at but all I can see are mounds of gauze. They tell me the incisions look great. *Uggg. I don't want to be here. I want to fast forward through this part please.*

I try to drink a bunch of water but am clearly too ambitious, as it all comes back up not long after. I try to get up and walk but end up throwing up again in a garbage can in the hallway. This may take longer than I planned. I can always stay another night if I am not tolerating liquids. But as the morning goes on I start feeling more alive and every hour seems to make a difference in my recovery. By the early afternoon I am eating soup and walking stiffly around the wards. I watch a TV show about a guy trapped in a volcano for three days and think how I at least am better off than that guy. By 4 PM I am dressed and eager to leave.

Before I go, the surgery team comes back to do their afternoon rounds. They all look so chipper still, but I can now match their collective mood better. One of them tells me he is the husband of one of my pathology residents. Now there's a nice team, a surgeon who removes things and a pathologist who tells him what it is. They wish me well and head off. But one medical student, who had introduced himself to me earlier in the pre-OP area, stays behind. He tells me how he was in the medical school class I lectured to on breast cancer pathology back in May when I was first undergoing chemotherapy. He tells me how much my lecture impacted him and that he hopes that I keep giving it to subsequent classes. I tell him I am planning on it.

It is pouring rain outside as I clamor cautiously up into Ryan's truck, trying hard not to flex my pectoral muscles at all, which are now tenderly stretched over my implants. We drive home uneventfully and Ryan fixes me some buttered noodles for dinner. The house is perfectly quiet except for the dog since the kids are with my parents for the week. I can't imagine how I could face the kids right now and am really glad that I have some time on my own to recover. We set up camp in our bedroom and watch the Sex in the City movie On-Demand. There's nothing like watching those four fashion-crazed women making messes of their lives to take your mind off our own! I sleep well that night, flat on my back, in my own bed again. The pain is really not that bad as long as I am not moving around too much.

The hardest part is over now, I tell myself.

Waiting for Pathology

T HE HARDEST PART IS over, but a few days after the surgery I am eagerly awaiting my pathology results. My MRI had shown such a great response, and I really want to know if my pathology matches those results. That is part of what I love about the field of pathology—it is the final say, the diagnosis that everything is based off of. And here I am waiting for my own pathology. Now I know how anxious patients feel while waiting for my report. I try to be patient and follow my own advice to those seeking preliminary results, *do you want the quick answer or the right answer?*

I have seen many a breast cancer case with specks of residual cancer scattered throughout a large, scarred area after being treated with chemotherapy and having a good response by imaging and that is not going to cut the mustard for me. I want a *complete* pathologic response, meaning not a single group of residual carcinoma cells hanging out resisting therapy. I am a perfectionist, and I want the A+. I have believed in my chemotherapy and have been imagining the cancer evaporating every day, but I also saw the ugly cancer that was still there after three months of Adriamycin and Cytoxan, so doubt is not far from the surface of my mind.

If it is gone completely, I will not need the additional three months of chemotherapy that the trial I am on requires. Even better than that, most studies have shown much better overall survival in patients who achieve a complete pathologic response. We are talking about long-term survival, here. I *really* want to be in that camp, but I remind myself that only the minority gets such a complete response, and even then, there is no guarantee it will never come back.

I know that I may hear my results today, so I try hard not to think about it too much. Good things come to those who wait, and it *will* be good things. It *better* be.

Around 2:00 PM the phone call comes, and my favorite surgeon in the world tells me . . . drumroll, please . . . there is *nothing* left: no invasive cancer in the breast and none in the lymph nodes.

Nothing.

Nada.

All gone.

I feel saved.

I stand up and shout.

I am Fraulein Maria from *The Sound of Music,* spinning with my arms outstretched on a green hilltop and singing at the top of my lungs.

I can hardly absorb it all. I see a bright, renewed future ahead of me. I am there when my kids graduate from college and to meet my grandkids. I could grow old with Ryan. I know this is still no guarantee of a long life—no one really ever has that—but I am so grateful to not be fighting the statistics of the poor survival group. I am so thankful for this experience and to have this end result. I am so grateful to be treated in this day and age where we can get this kind of response to aggressive forms of cancer. I know exactly what this means: I am one lucky lady.

The Unveiling

A FEW DAYS AFTER SURGERY, it is time to take the bandages off. I stand in front of the mirror and tear open the Velcro bra. A thick tape is covering my upper chest to try and "keep the implants medial" (i.e., give me a little cleavage for the first time in my life!). Ryan cuts through this, releasing the tension, and immediately I can breathe easier. Underneath the tape, my skin is all wrinkled and molded from the creases in the bandage, but there are two decent-sized mounds of breast-like tissue there. They really are shaped like Barbie's boobs. Smooth, hard, nipple-less "lady lumps" that sit up unnaturally high. There is more gauze to remove from the chest area and under my armpits where the drains are exiting out little holes in the skin. A tiny suture holds each drain in place. When we finally have peeled everything away, I feel amazingly lighter. The skin over my new breasts is pretty numb; it must be the stretched pectoralis muscle beneath the implant that causes the burning I feel if I move funny.

I take a look in the mirror at the new bionic me. They look to be an ample B cup—maybe even a light C—quite perky but still a bit lumpy from all the bandaging. There are horizontal scars running across the area where my nipples once were, but they are very neatly sewn with clear sutures. *Yes, the new ones will do just fine.* Ryan, who was a little freaked out by all the slow tape removal, also seems satisfied with the results. *Great! I'll take 'em.* Hopefully, radiation will treat them gently and not cause them to contract and need replacement too soon.

Ryan and I lie low for several days. I like being holed up in my little pain cave with him. We watch movies, play backgammon, and stay cozy. I have very little desire to talk with anyone else. We do venture out a few times a day to eat or run an errand. I pin my drains up under my shirt to hide them. Let me tell you: these drains do little for fashion. Under my sweater, they look like extra lumps of fat hanging off my sides, and if I am not careful, the long loops of tubing sometimes peek out from the bottom of my shirt. Plus I am walking like an eighty-year old now—a bit hunched over and taking delicate, deliberate steps. I have traded my Velcro bra, which was getting itchy and tight, for a belly-band I used during pregnancy, and it works perfectly as a strapless, soft camisole that I could step into. I just could not bring myself to buy one of those official post-mastectomy bras for some reason, although I am sure they are convenient, too. I did buy a fabulous hospital gown of sorts that really looks more like a cross between a kimono and an Asian-style jacket (www.healingthreads.com). It was not exactly cheap, but it was perfect to wear for the first several days because not only does it bear no resemblance to an actual hospital gown, it has all sorts of Velcro access panels *and* pockets for drains. Why not attempt to look a little bit fabulous while convalescing? I can wear it out of the house and people have no idea of what lies beneath. But after several days in the same getup, I get tired of this, too. Right now, anything from my closet that has to be pulled over my head seems off-limits.

One afternoon during the first week, I feel up for joining Ryan on our monthly sojourn to acquire mass quantities of diapers from Costco. As I enter the giant superstore, I am smuggling my drains around like little hams under my sweater. I am waiting for someone to suspect I am shoplifting and ask me, "Ma'am, excuse me, but what is under that sweater?" I secretly want someone to, so I can see the horrified look on his or her face when I say "I understand," and unzip the sweater to reveal the bloody drain bombs dangling from the inside of my sweater. I am so cruel. But no one bats an eye. They probably just think I'm a lumpy-looking lady.

After a week or two, my drains have stopped putting out much fluid. Once they stop putting out a certain amount I can get them removed, so I have been keeping a close score in a "drain diary."

Dear Drain Diary,

Today you made 30cc of yellow-red fluid that did not have a foul odor. You also stayed nicely pinned under my shirt without trying to peek at the world. It was a good day.

Back to the Real World

IT IS A SUNNY fall day, with colors so bright outside it makes my eyes hurt. I think of all the cones in my retina that are firing as my pupils dilate to take in the image of a bright yellow tree. Why is it that right before their retirement, leaves burn with such intense hues? I feel like they are vibrating around me, creating a symphony of color in celebration of my cancer-free existence. Sometimes when I am driving alone in my car surrounded by the fireworks of fall I just scream at the top of my lungs, *THANK YOU!* And then I smile at whoever is next to me at the stoplight. But my journey is not over yet. I still have radiation, another nine months of IV Herceptin antibody therapy, nipple reconstruction (plus that crazy areola tattoo) and all that business of *survival* to get to. For now though, I am still swimming in my success and quietly recovering treatment-free.

I am sitting in my backyard swinging gently on a porch swing listening to the silence I so rarely hear with two small kids usually underfoot. The calm is occasionally punctuated by a crow balking. I am relaxed—sore but relaxed. No more stress about getting sick before my OR date. No more concerns about whether there will be cancer left or the possibility of more chemotherapy. Ryan is waiting on me hand and foot (I could really get used to this!). I am in a peaceful place.

I hear a little girl calling for her mother from the neighbor's backyard and I feel a heartstring tug inside me. I have been so content in my post-OP peace, with just Ryan and I, our biggest worry being what to eat for dinner. Hearing the little girl reminds me of Maddy, and now I am picturing what she and Henry would be doing right now if they were here. Henry would clearly be climbing up on something or marching around with two identical items in each hand, chattering away in his adorably unintelligible style. Maddy would be offering me tea made of water and flower petals and then floating around the pavement on her pink bicycle, her long stork-like legs slowly pumping. She would be singing a wistful song, lost in her imaginary scenarios, my little drama queen. When she was only two, she used to wander around the house singing "Ohhh I've seen everything, I've seen everything . . ." with a wistful look on her face. She practices crying in the mirror. (I am *not* looking forward to the teenage years!). I am a mother-hen without her chicks. I realize I am getting ready to leave my peaceful zone and re-enter the chaos of life.

But it also feels like things have shifted in my world. Henry will return saying a few new more intelligible words. Maddy will have learned a new song from the latest Disney movie. We will even have a new president of the country soon. And I have new (still nippleless) breasts. But it is really more than that. I feel like I have been gently placed back upon the Earth after being uprooted and hosed off with cold water and now I am supposed to find a new path or rediscover the old one I was on. *What is the next step? Back to the same old ways?*

What Is the New Normal?

I AM FEELING GOOD NOW, about three and half weeks out from surgery. The kids came back two weeks ago and Maddy has been fantastic about not asking me to lift her up and being careful about my "boobie surgery." Henry had a little trouble with the concept of not being in my arms whenever he asked but I spent a lot of time kneeling on the floor to be close to him. He is getting more self-sufficient now at fifteen months. You can tell him to go put his shoes on to go and he actually does it. I had my mother around again for a bit to help out and Ryan and Halia continued to haul Henry around once she left. I have to say I enjoyed not having to wrestle him on the changing table for a while. But now I am picking him up without any pain. In fact, I am feeling physically pretty close to normal again. My right underarm is still really numb and sensitive from the axillary dissection and I still feel really "tight" and can't lift my arms up all the way above my head but all in all I am back doing most of what I could do before surgery.

It is the night after Halloween and Ryan and I are getting ready to go to a costume party. I am excited about my costume and looking forward to seeing a lot of people I haven't seen in ages—some not since "B.C." (Before Cancer). I wanted my costume to play off my super-short hair, which is basically a fuzzy crew cut at this point. I thought about being Peter Pan or a Buddhist monk but finally decided to go with a "gruntie" or freshman rower since I already had all the gear from Opening Day. The shaved head look would work perfectly with that theme and then Ryan could dress as our friend the UW varsity rowing coach, Mike Callahan. Ryan hates dressing up for Halloween, but he is actually excited about our idea and is strutting around in bright orange foul-weather gear borrowed from Coach Callahan's launch boat. He really looks the part when he adds a stopwatch, megaphone, UW cap, and glasses to the ensemble. I am wearing a Freshman Rowing t-shirt, spandex, and my running shoes.

"Don't you think I should be more obvious about who I am? Maybe a sign that says, 'Gruntie'?" I ask Ryan as I check myself out in the mirror.

"No, no. You're perfect. Everyone will know what you are, it is so obvious," he answers.

"It's not obvious if you weren't a rower," I answer. "I don't know. Maybe I should be something a little more sexy. I could show off my new hooters a bit more."

"No you look great Kim. It's perfect."

I decide I don't really care too much how I look but I do bother to put lipstick on. And at least the costume is comfortable. I'd wear the same thing to workout.

We load ourselves into my car and race off to our first grown-up party since we can't remember when. We turn the music up and sing Coldplay as we race through the streets with high spirits. There are supposed to be over a hundred people at the party. Costumes are mandatory. It's time for some fun!

"OK Ry-guy, just remember to stick with me. My costume doesn't really make sense without you next to me." I remind Ryan as we walk up to the open door.

We step into the house and immediately I realize I have made a mistake. There is the hostess in a beautiful sexy white dress, dolled up as Cleopatra with golden bands and strappy shoes. I have forgotten the cardinal rule of Halloween for females: it doesn't matter what your costume is, as long as you *look* good. I should have learned my lesson after that Halloween in New York City when I was in medical school and Ryan and I went as Vikings draped in shapeless bolts of faux fur. That night I watched my girlfriends, who were all dressed in tight black outfits from no particular genre, wiggling around the dance floor in their slinky get-ups. There is no dancing sexy as a female Viking.

So the hostess is happy to see me but I can tell that she has no idea what I am supposed to be dressed as and maybe thinks I literally did just come from the gym. I turn to find Ryan and he is already gone.

The party starts to swallow me up. I am surrounded by strangers in bizarre costumes and I don't recognize a soul. Finally I find my friend Jessica, who looks gorgeous dressed as a witch in a low-cut black dress. She starts introducing me to friends and I end up explaining to people I've just met that no, I didn't shave my head for my costume, I just went through six months of chemotherapy. But everything's fine now. Yes, nice to meet you too.

I am a buzz-kill. I am the cancer-kid.

More people I know begin to show up and recognize me. They hug me and tell me how good it is to see me. They tell me they have been reading my blog. Some of them are people I barely know and I am wondering how they found out about my online diary and am trying to remember how many embarrassing details I have posted. Everyone is very serious with me. They want to know how I am doing and how I have coped. I try to say a joke about my new boobs and no one laughs.

Crap, I am supposed to be having fun and I am feeling totally disconnected to the party atmosphere around me. People ask me if I am drinking again because I am holding a glass of wine. I can't even enjoy half a glass before I begin to feel too guilty about it and set it down again. It is getting really loud and I can barely understand what people are saying anymore so I give up and stand quietly by the buffet table. I feel like I am just watching everyone have a great time without me. For the first time, I am looking around the room of 30-to-40- somethings and wondering, *of all these people,* why me?

Why do I have to be scarred by this? I feel like I am wearing a pink ribbon like a scarlet letter.

Then the "entertainment" shows up. A topless woman with her skin painted a corpse-like white leaps up onto the buffet centerpiece, which is shaped like a coffin. She lies down as another woman decorates her with drips and slashes of a thick blood-colored fluid. Then she clutches a bouquet of dead black roses to her chest and lies still in her coffin next to the platters of salami and cheese. They have really spiced things up, but it also seems strangely tasteful, like performance art. The men are all staring at her naked chest in awe. They probably haven't seen anything like this since their fraternity days.

I am staring at her perfect, real nipples with envy.

I don't belong here. I look for Ryan and tell him I want to leave. He sees the look in my eyes, puts down his beer and we head for the door.

My First Tattoo

I AM LYING ON A table with my left arm arched over my head, my hand grasping a metal bar. I am cradled in a warm mold of my upper body, which the radiation technologists have just made by mixing two compounds together to make a foam. I pass in and out of a CT scan machine while the technologists chat with me.

"So do I get to keep my body mold when I am done with therapy?" I ask them as I eye a nearby shelf full of wrapped molds labeled with patients' names.

"Yes! That will be your personal radiation therapy souvenir," one of them quips.

I try to imagine what I would do with a used half-body mold. Use it as a boogie board? Would it float? Mount it on the wall at home somewhere as a misshapen piece of modern art? Give it to my kids to use as a racecar track?

My left hand is going painfully numb from being held over my head for so long.

"I really have to move my arm," I say hopefully.

"Sit tight, we are almost through."

My doctor re-checks my position and my scans. All is to her liking so they start marking me up with pens. Dotted lines and targets cross my chest like a treasure map. I can finally let my arm down and my fingers burn with the reawakening of my nerves.

Then I get my first tattoo: four tiny black dots in different areas across my upper body, made by placing ink on my skin and then pricking me with a needle. I jump each time. How do people stand the big tattoo procedures? How am I going to deal with the whole areola tattoo that awaits me in my reconstruction future?

I look down at my tattoos. They look like little black freckles or like I accidentally stuck myself with a black ballpoint pen. I proudly display my tiny "tats" to Ryan. I tell him that they actually say his name in tiny micro-writing, like they engrave on diamonds. He knows I'm kidding. I need to try this one on someone more gullible. My mother falls for it hook, line, and sinker and is honored one says "mom," until I reveal the joke.

The thought of six weeks of radiation five days a week is not enticing at all right now. I feel like I made it through the woods already with chemotherapy and surgery behind me. I am four weeks out from surgery now and getting my mobility back. My left armpit was initially tight from the axillary dissection. I could barely lift my arm at first, but now I can lift it all the way above my shoulders again. The skin over my chest is still under a lot of tension though and I don't really want to stress it more with radiation. Plus I had such a great response to the chemotherapy—do I really need this therapeutic sunburn? The reality of another stage in my treatment is tiring. I don't want any more doctors' appointments. I have even been skipping out on acupuncture because I am just tired of having so many health related appointments. *Can't I just go on with life? I did it. The cancer is gone.* I feel like a sick little kid asking her mom, *"Come on can't I PLEASE go out to play?"*

But it has always been the plan to have radiation therapy. Radiation is local therapy usually only given to breast cancer patients after a lumpectomy. The idea is that the radiation kills off any possible remaining diving cells after surgery to reduce your risk of local recurrence. Usually choosing a mastectomy will minimize the chance of any residual microscopic disease so much that radiation is not necessary. But in cases that are particularly large (> 5 cm) or have other high-risk features like an inflammatory cancer, radiation has been shown to reduce local recurrences to the chest wall after mastectomy too. I have done my homework and know that even with a complete response to chemotherapy, like I had, radiation may still help prevent a local recurrence. I should be a good patient and take my medicine. At least radiation is a local therapy that won't affect my whole body since it is being delivered to only my left chest area. It should really be the easiest part of my therapy so far.

They will take another week or two to "make a plan." What do they mean by "make a plan?" Can't I just sign up for a time slot to get my rays like at a tanning salon? What is there to plan? Apparently, they work out a whole simulation of the way that my radiation will be targeted on my particular body using my CT images. A physicist actually goes over the whole plan to make sure that the correct zones are targeted with minimal effects on other vital organs like my heart and lungs. I will have to be carefully positioned back in my body mold each time so that the identical area is treated. This is clearly more sophisticated than just going to a tanning bed for some photons.

I really don't want this part of therapy to get me down. I feel like I am just coming out of the wilderness and finding parts of my old life strewn like garbage on the side of the road. I pick up a piece, examine it and have to decide if it is worth keeping or not. I have started gingerly running again, which has brought back a whole flood of memories. I was training for my first half-marathon when I was diagnosed. I never made it to the finish line of that race and I wonder if I will ever have the courage to try for that goal again. I feel like whatever I was doing before had to be wrong in some way since I ended up with cancer. If I tried again would I have a recurrence? It sounds so silly and superstitious. Exercise is supposed to *prevent* cancer. And it does feel great to get that exercise buzz again. I love the solitude of running and being outside to take in the natural world around me. I do notice new things now, like how the tops of the pine trees along my route have been twisted and bent by the environment around them. Nature is as imperfect and adaptive as me. But even listening to the same songs I used to run to also seems so strange, like trying to place myself in a time that seems distant and discordant with today. I make a new mix of songs to run to with titles like Alicia Keys' "Superwoman". Because I deserve to feel like I have some superpowers after all this.

Five Weeks of Sunburn

MY RADIATION PLAN GETS finalized and I am called back in for some final X-rays to set up the exact radiation fields I will be getting. They make a custom-fit piece of smoky yellow material to place over my left chest to enhance treatment of the skin, where most post-mastectomy recurrences develop. It is called a bolus. I ask the techs what it is made of. They are not sure exactly but they say it is called "Superflab." *You've got to be kidding me. Superflab?* It sounds like Flubber from that old Disney movie, *The Absent Minded Professor.* My Flubber-shield will be draped over my left bionic breast throughout treatment.

My first day of treatment I drive reluctantly to the cancer center. I *really* don't want to go. If I were my daughter I would be crying and screeching "I don't wanna go! I don't wanna go! PLEASE don't make me go!"

It's not that I think it will hurt, although I am worried about my sensitive skin. I just don't want to go through one more phase of treatment. And this one is daily. I am feeling tired of doctors' appointments. And I don't want to ruin my perfectly good implant and have to have another surgery because of radiation damage.

I am on time for my 8:45 AM time slot. A woman with shoulder-length blonde hair gets called in ahead of me. As I am changing into a gown I hear a recording go off in the treatment room and a tinny song erupts, "Celebrate good times . . . come on!" *How can they be having so much fun in there?*

The door opens and the woman ahead of me is leaving, gown askew, with a big grin on her face.

"Congrats on your last treatment," the tech tells her as she waltzes out.

And here I go, Day One.

They call me in and I lie down on the table, which is covered by a warm blanket. Frank Sinatra is playing in the background. I sink into my mold, left arm raised and head turned to the right towards the large gyroscope-like machine positioned to the side of the table. I stare into the crosshairs of the target as the techs busy themselves around me. They tug on the sheet beneath me adjusting me slightly one way, then another. They call out coordinates to each other.

"98.5"

"Check"

"101.3"

"OK"

"B11"

"You sunk my battleship!" I quip. *Have they heard this joke before? Because they aren't really laughing.*

They put in place my Flubber-shield. Then they leave the room quickly for my 30-second dose. The machine makes cooing noises as I lie still and try to tell myself, *This is making me stronger. This is making me stronger.*

I feel absolutely nothing as the radiation is silently delivered. Then the techs return and recheck coordinates as they adjust the machine to treat the next field. The gyroscope turns towards my armpit. They leave the room and I get my "alone-time" with the machine again. Quiet photons pass through the Flubber-shield.

For the third and final field they remove the Flubber-shield and the crosshairs line up to target the area around my clavicle (where the supraclavicular lymph nodes hide). Again, I am alone with the machine, breasts exposed with Frank Sinatra playing. I am a very still dance partner. I am being wooed by an android.

The second week of radiation, a professorial man with white

hair and a mustache enters the treatment room. The techs tell me he is the department physicist. He checks the numbers and computer simulations of where the radiation is being targeted. *How cool, my own personal physicist.* I shake his hand eagerly and start asking him questions. He tells me about things like the machine's tungsten fingers that curl and uncurl to alter the radiation fields. How romantic—tungsten fingers . . .

Eventually, he asks if I would like to see the rest of the machine. I feel like Dorothy about to meet the Wizard of OZ as he leads me to a little door adjacent to where the machine is mounted on the wall. We step into a dim room dominated by a mammoth of a creature. Unlike its slick counterpart on the other side of the wall, this side is raw and exposed with patches of loosely organized wires hanging like guts off its sides. I am amazed that such a beast can deliver such targeted delicate photons. I get a short lesson that I struggle to comprehend and then we resurface on the other side. The wizard shakes my hand and disappears to his calculations.

I get to know my technologists well and we start having fun together. I ask them what they named their machine, thinking like good techies they would have come up with some android name for the linear accelerator. Apparently the poor guy was nameless so we decide to dub him something from *Star Wars* and what better gentleman android is there than C3PO? As I finish treatment that day suddenly the *Star Wars* soundtrack is playing over the loudspeaker. I really like these guys.

Every day I am greeted by C3PO and an ever changing daily music dose. Instead of elevator music, these techs clearly have more youthful taste in music and have created personal CDs for the treatment room ambiance. Day 1 is Lenny Kravitz. Day 2 is Jamiroquai. Day 3 is the *Forrest Gump* soundtrack. Day 4 is Sara McLachlan. Day 5 is John Mayer. Day 6 Boy George, "Do you really want to hurt me?" Day 7 is Jack Johnson. The hits continue and the whole process becomes like a routine dance. I come in and lie down in my dance position with my left arm raised above my head like I am about to samba. C3PO spins his arm around me and curls his tungsten fingers to the music. I lie still and wink at him as he romances me with several long beeps and the dance is over.

Overall, I find the whole five weeks of radiation treatment relatively non-toxic. The daily visits and scheduling the rest of life around them do wear on me and I hate not being able to drive my daughter to school because my standing appointment is at the same time as school drop-off. But she takes this in stride, the now-adaptable five-year old. The vision I had of a frighteningly archaic dinosaur of a machine zapping me and sapping all my energy did not come to fruition. And my skin and implants are doing fine as I approach the final fifth week.

My last week, the field is narrowed to my scar only for a "boost" of electrons instead of photons (most local recurrences actually occur along the scar line). This treatment is even faster, but I have a big ink rectangle drawn around my scar with permanent marker for the week. I also develop an incredibly itchy rash across my abdomen that perplexes the nurses and physicians that see it. They don't want me to blame them since it is not confined to the radiation field—they say it's more likely an allergy to something—but maybe I have just developed a whole body allergy to radiation . . . It drives me mad not to be able to itch it because I don't want to break down any skin in the radiated area. But a little Benadryl, cortisone cream, and time and it disappears.

The last week of radiation is a week of major snow storms in the Seattle area that literally shut the city down. Seattle-ites are used to rain, not snow, and the hilly urban streets become completely impassible sheets of ice and chunky snow. There are not enough snow plows and apparently for environmental reasons they don't even use salt on the roads. Back east where I went to college and medical school, this storm wouldn't have slowed anyone down. But here, inexperienced drivers in two-wheel drive sports cars are sliding all over the roads, making the actual drivers themselves even more hazardous than the snow and ice. Winter break comes early for schools as they shut down and offices go to essential staff only. Ryan's restaurant/wine shop is silent the week before Christmas, which is supposed to be the very peak of his sales season. The whole nation seems in a similar state of disaster with spiraling stock markets, bail outs and general economic malaise. 2008 is going out with a fight and I am looking forward to the promises of recovery in 2009.

I skip a day of radiation and play in the snow with my kids. Maddy is finally old enough to tolerate snow play for long enough to get in some good sledding and build a decent snow man. Henry wanders stiffly in his puffy snowsuit and cries each time he falls down but still wants in on the action. We have no choice but to enjoy ourselves and be together—like a big white blessing. I do manage to get to radiation for my final few treatments before we head off to the Bay Area to be with my family for the holidays. On my last day of radiation they play me the same "Celebrate Good Times" song I heard played for someone else on my first day of treatment. I do a little dance, hand them a music CD I made for them and say my good-byes to C3PO. I am done and I feel not much worse for the wear.

It is not until the week after finishing treatment—Christmas week—that my skin finally revolts.

How dare you treat me like this! My skin screams with angry red patches formed in the general outline of a triangle from the radiation field. Burned brown scales and tiny blisters appear in clusters. They begin to lift off and peel, leaving raw, virgin skin exposed. It oozes and crusts, constantly weeping a creepy yellow goo which gets all over whatever I am wearing. My chest looks like a mosaic of red, yellow, and brown layers of pain. It all seems so wrong to be corroding away like this when I am supposed to be done with therapy. It somehow seems worse than all the surgery and the chemo because I am no longer bracing myself to weather the awfulness of it all. I whine and wallow my way through.

It hurts to wear clothes. It hurts to move my arm. It hurts to move in bed. I want to burn off my holiday splurge calories but the thought of putting on an athletic bra makes me hurt as well and keeps me idle. I was not expecting this, which makes it all the worse. And it keeps getting worse. Eventually, the entire area is an oozing open wound.

After I get back from my Christmas vacation I go see my radiation oncologist.

"Does this happen to everyone?" I ask a bit confrontationally as I lift my shirt and bear my wounds.

"Well, radiation affects everyone differently. Most people don't but some people peel like you are." The nurse answers calmly as she examines my mosaic of raw skin.

"Peel" like me?

This is beyond peeling, this is ulcerating.

I still feel like this can't possibly be normal. So many women get radiation post-lumpectomy and the vast majority of them don't get this kind of reaction. I guess with the relative lack of complications from chemotherapy and surgery, it is now my time to get the short end of the stick.

She gives me some Silvadene cream, which I remember is used on burn patients to keep from getting infections. She has me spackle my chest with the thick white cream and covers the area with non-stick dressings. Then she has me slip into a white fishnet tube-top to wear so the dressings stay in place. This does feel more comfortable. It is strange how unlike when on chemotherapy, where you have more obvious external signs of going through something serious, now with radiation burns they are hidden quietly under my bandages and shirt so no one sees the pain. People keep congratulating me on being done with treatment. I wish I could lift my shirt in response and say, "You think I'm *done* dealing with this?"

But I have come a long way now. I look in the mirror one morning after finishing all my bandaging and take a long hard look at my reflection. My hair has grown back to a good inch and a half. I hardly recognize myself in the mirror with my spiky version of the Audrey Hepburn pixie cut. I am trying on a new me. When I look back at photographs from "before," I look so young with my blonde pony tail perched on the back of my head. My hair has always been thin and fine without much body. But now with it so short, it actually looks thick and has a bit of curl to it. I look a bit like a labradoodle, with some sort of hybrid puffy, curly, wavy hair. I stare carefully at myself in the mirror, evaluating this newcomer. I think I like the newer, wiser me. I look well traveled and grown up. People I know that haven't seen me for a while walk right past me without recognizing me. I am a secret agent cruising through my old life in a new disguise.

Desert Renewal

MY SKIN EVENTUALLY TURNS a corner after a few weeks
of ulcerating. New mottled reddish skin has populated all but
one patch and I am down to wearing only one bandage, without the
silly mesh top. Just in time too. My angel of a mother had invited me
to a spa in the warm desert of Arizona for some rejuvenation. God
bless her. I could not have created a better mother if I had hand-picked
her. We jive. We run on the same frequency. We used to be able to
guess what number the other was thinking when I was little, a talent
we lost as I grew older. And even though I ended up with some very
different traits than her, we always felt more like sisters than mother
and daughter. Some good mother-daughter time would be nice. Not
to mention the warm weather and all the spa accoutrements.

I cherish the solitude of the toddler-free plane ride to Tucson. It
is so nice to focus only on myself for a change while flying. I thrive
in the solitude. I play on my laptop and actually read a bit of a novel.
When I land and head to baggage claim, I quickly spot my mother's
straw and chestnut hairdo and brightly colored jacket at the baggage
claim. We excitedly chatter about the days ahead and roll our bags
outside into the warm night air. A shuttle takes us to our airport
hotel for the night and we spend a restless evening in-between before
we head to our final destination.

We arrive the next morning and are unleashed on the spa territory. We explore frantically, disoriented to this other slow-paced
world.

"What hikes should we sign up for?"

"What treatments should we be getting?"

"What meals should we be eating and where?"

And most importantly, "Where the heck is our room?"

The place is so understated that we can't even find the labels on the buildings and we spend the first few hours trying to figure out how all the curved pathways connect.

We try a yoga class and still cannot unwind. Finally we both have our first heavenly treatment. It is called a warm vanilla float. I had picked it out of the catalogue since the name made me absolutely drool. This is our turning point—like a christening into our peaceful experience.

We robe up in the spa locker rooms and pass through a room with a series of hot pools on our way to the treatment waiting area. Two naked women are bubbling away in the hot tubs, their bare breasts floating on the surface foam. I self-consciously cling to the nipple-less mounds under my robe and make a mental note to schedule my nipple reconstruction surgery.

When my name is called in the waiting area they lead me to a dark hallway of doors and then to my candlelit room. I am told to undress and lie on a blanketed table. The therapist slowly rubs a loufa over my skin, rubbing off the dry and tired layers. I am told to take a shower in a chamber full of jets spraying at me from many directions. Then I am led to a different table covered by a warm sheet. I sit on the cold edge and begin to be slathered in thick layers of buttery vanilla-scented lotion. I lay back on the table and another warm sheet is layered on top of me. Then the bottom of the table begins to lower and I find myself suspended in a hammock created by a warm waterbed. I rock and wiggle with a smile on my face and sink into the womb that has formed around me. Hmmmm . . . the real world has melted away as I float into vanilla-scented bliss. When I emerge, my skin is thicker and softer and I have finally succeeded in slowing down to a relaxed spa-pace. My mother, who just had the same treatment an hour earlier, and I float on our vanilla clouds to dinner.

The rest of our time we spend going on hikes through the desert, trying new classes and eating healthy but delicious meals. I try an underwater massage called "watsu," a world beat dance class, a clairvoyant reading and "healing touch". We meet new people and none of them know my history unless I volunteer it. Too quickly the last night approaches.

I slip away for a little reflection. I feel drawn away, toward the landscape beyond the compound. I pass the rust colored buildings, the tennis courts and swimming pool and find my way to a sandy path leading off into the desert. The sun is dipping towards the horizon and the sky is painted a clear gentle blue offset by strips of orange clouds. The wind is picking up, arriving like a mysterious visitor, it twists and moves about the dry landscape. I can hear it before it catches me and whispers warm magic across my cheek.

There is a dry peace about the desert. I take in the slow twist of a barrel cactus that I pass on the dusty trail. I watch the vibration and stillness of the ancient saguro cactus. Hundreds of years old, they stand like tall ancestors, arms pointed upwards or outstretched in slow gestures. I imagine I can hear an electric hum emanating from them. I reach out to touch one, careful to avoid the lines of thorns running up its sides like spines. I am surprised by its turgor—this water-filled stalk seems to push back into my fingertips with smooth strength. I wink at the ones that have lost a limb or are carved with many woodpecker holes and still stand tall and strong. They are survivors too.

I reach a flat labyrinth made of many white stones and pace through its twisted loops. At the center is a small shrine of stones and various items that others have left behind. A brown crystal, a green wristband, a pink ribbon, a packet of iodized salt (something someone has decided to give up?). I run my eyes over my hands and arms searching for something to leave. With nothing of significance on hand I lean forward and let a thin strand of saliva slip from my mouth like a silvery web. It leaves a wet mark on one of the dusty rocks in the pile and I am satisfied with my biological contribution.

I turn and wind my way back to another path lined by more white stones. This one leads to a narrow teepee, its sides partially covered in patches of cloth and windings of yarn and ribbon. I duck inside and a shower of messages dangling from bits of yarn are landing on my head and shoulders. I stoop between them, smiling and clasping at the twinkling surprises. Some are objects like crystals or seed pods. Others are bits of paper with messages. I turn the papers over to read their secrets. "I will love myself," one reads. "For Jesse," reads another. Some are washed blank by time and weather but they still hang with the same intention. They are such personal messages, like peering into the deepest parts of someone's heart. But surrounded by them I feel like I am in a space full of my own supporters—fellow humans with struggles and secrets and pains and beauty that link us all. I hold their hands in that narrow teepee and we embrace each other, for a moment protected from the glorious uncertainty of the world outside the enclosure.

I climb a small side trail that is marked by a large rounded stone engraved with the word *spirit*. Visitors before me have contributed to an irregular pyramid of smaller rocks atop this large one. Like spiritual, nameless graffiti, marking that they were here too and found some grace in this spot. I balance a flat red stone on the top. I was here too. More engraved rocks sit crouched along the path up the hill like trolls, each with their own hats of collectively piled stones. Tibetan prayer flags wag quietly from a few of the dry bushes. At the top of the hill the landscape unrolls before me. The flat desert floor is broken only by the evenly-spaced Saguro, which form thousands of sage-colored pillars across the dry plane. The surrounding mountains jut up suddenly, pushing the horizon upwards abruptly into spotted folds of earth peaked by rectangular faces of bare rock.

It is the golden hour. That time when the sun is making its nest at the edge of the sky and emanating a final subdued candlelight that makes the spot of the Earth it is slipping past absolutely glow. The atmosphere becomes heavy with a thicker, softer light made of pure melted butter. I drink in the still air. I am at peace.

Happy Cancer-Versary

T HE EARTH HAS MADE one complete revolution around the hot red sun. The stars and planets have repositioned themselves in relation to my spot in the universe so that I am re-aligned with the way they were exactly one year ago. The weather is similar, with cold March mornings and rainy afternoons. Spring flowers are attempting to emerge from the chill wet earth and the sunlight is beginning to linger longer at the end of the day.

Today is my cancer-versary.

One year and one day ago I was happily nursing my baby boy completely oblivious to the storm brewing inside me. Then one year ago today, I received the lightning bolt shock of a cancer diagnosis. Hard to believe the lifetime I have experienced since then has only been encompassed by a single year.

All that water under my bridge—the emotion of the first few weeks feeling like my life had ended, the long road through chemotherapy, the second hit of surgery, and the third whammy of radiation—and of course, the joy of having a good response to therapy, reducing (but not eliminating) my worries about a recurrence. But somehow, bringing time back full circle has filled my head once again with thoughts of cancer and its sneaky ugly ways. Like getting closer to the abyss again, only since I have seen it before it is not nearly as terrifying. I try to bounce the energy away, keep myself protected, keep the bad thoughts out but they seem to settle in like little cats curling up for long evening naps. I realize these worries will never be far from the surface and so I invite them to stay a while and listen to their terrible purring. I stay busy bouncing through cluttered work days and whirlwind evenings of kids and dinner and bathtime and bedtime, thinking the slow purr will be drowned out. Only if I pause, if I am finally still, I can hear them again whispering my concerns. But I also realize how comfortable I have become with these thoughts so they are actually no longer really fears but little possible truths that I turn over in my mind again and again until they are smooth and round and shiny and digested.

One year ago I was completely enveloped in fear, literally shaking like a wounded bird waiting for everything to come apart. But I let go and believed in my treatment, in myself, and in seeing the world as a magical place where good things can happen. (My friend Claudia is convinced that my cancer is gone through 97% medical treatment and 3% magic.) And now, having weathered a storm I was terrified to travel through, I can see how much stronger and at peace I have become. I feel like a great energy was born in me and it continues to glow.

Like red sunshine.

Note to Co-Survivors

I FEEL INCREDIBLY LUCKY TO have learned so much through my experience with breast cancer both as a patient and as a physician. If you have recently been touched by this disease I am sure you have heard lots of different advice already. Here is my short list of mantras/advice—take it or leave it! I wish you strength and insight on your journey.

- Keep *LIVING*—whether you have been told your prognosis is excellent or guarded, you are here *now* and very much alive
- Believe in your treatment and your treatment team
- Educate yourself on your options—there can be lots of them
- Second opinions are always a good idea (not just on therapy options but on the pathology* and radiology as well)
- Let other people help and tell them *how* (most people have no clue!)
- Let go of the guilt: neither you nor the chocolate you ate did this
- Contact others who have a similar diagnosis
- Get fresh air every day and stay active
- Don't give up good distractions: keep working, volunteering, doing hobbies you love, etc., because you can't think about cancer *all* the time
- Embrace your new perspective—*The Big Picture*—and let the small stuff go

◆ Take this opportunity to put yourself first (you may not have a chance to be so selfish again!)

◆ Let the process change you for the better: this *will* make you stronger

*For more information on second opinions of your breast pathology by Dr. Allison, please see: www.pathology.washington.edu/clinical/breast

Afterword

W<small>RITING HAS ALWAYS BEEN</small> therapeutic for me. I was a
shy kid who wrote in my journal to sort through all my sen-
sitivities and imagine things like alternate universes and life without
braces. From grade school through medical school, writing was my
outlet as I tried to contemplate and digest where I was going and
what I was feeling. But somehow, as life got busier and my husband,
kids, and career needed more attention, I gave this up. Perhaps this
was a measure of my general happiness—I was no longer dreaming
about the life I could have because I was lucky enough to be *living* it.
But as soon as I was diagnosed with cancer, the desire to make sense
of my experience through writing was reborn with a new fervor. It
was amazing how, once my thoughts were put to words on a page
and reread, the experience suddenly became more enlightening as I
recognized both my strengths and weaknesses as well as the humor
and meaning in the process.

At first I was incredibly timid about sharing my writing with
others. The experience was too raw, emotional, and private to share
with anyone other than myself. But as time passed and I began to
emerge from the intensity, I realized that sharing my story might
be a brave, and perhaps necessary, thing to do. Other women who
were newly diagnosed began to contact me—just as I had contacted
others—looking for guidance and asking for a glimpse of what it was
like, wanting so badly to see that there could be light at the end of

the tunnel. And I realized that the more selfish act would be to keep this story to myself.

And so *Red Sunshine* was born. My hope is that my story will shed some light on dark times so that you can continue to shine in your own unique way. Whether you are a survivor of cancer or any other unexpected challenge, your reaction to an obstacle is always your choice. Be who you want to be . . . in this moment and always. Choose to see the magic in everyday experiences. Live wisely. And, as Lance Armstrong and his cohorts put it so well, *Live Strong*.

—*Kim*

For more information about Kim, and to continue following her on her journey, please visit www.redsunshine.org.

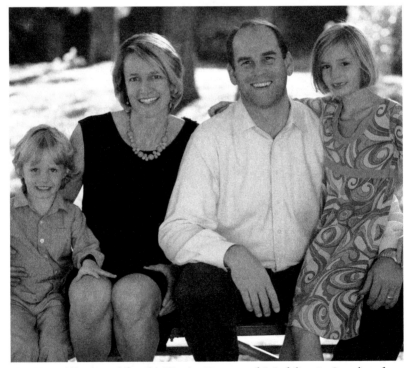

Dr. Kim Allison and family: Henry, Ryan, and Madeline in Seattle today.

Acknowledgments

I AM SO GRATEFUL TO all those who have supported me through this experience. Cancer can bring people together in amazing ways and give those affected an unexpected education that looking back, I now feel lucky to have received.

I owe my husband, Ryan, for giving me the support (although maybe *not* empathy!) and love I needed to feel like I was still a beautiful, young wife despite a cancer diagnosis. Today I actually miss the time we spent together on our "chemo dates." Our marriage is a survivor and is stronger for it. I also thank you for continuing to be such a fantastic father to our kids, Maddy and Henry.

I cannot thank the indefatigable "grandmothers," Emily and Gail, enough for all of their essential support. They truly amazed me with their rapid willingness to give up so much of their own lives to help keep mine together. The kids loved having you around so often. I loved all the home-cooked meals and great company. And if you don't mind, I am thinking we should probably keep it as at least a monthly re-union . . . I can only dream. I miss you.

Thank you to my father, Bob, who let my mother leave his side so many times to come take care of me. And thank you especially for reading my early manuscript and pushing me to get it out there. You are my truest advisor and always a believer in whatever I dream of doing.

Little brother, Chris, thanks for your willingness to show such solidarity. I am glad you never went full Monty on the head shaving. You look better with hair.

My colleagues at work were also amazingly supportive. From meals to service coverage, to having faith I would be able to continue working in my field, I am in debt to you. And to all the friends and supporters, "Thanks Team!" To those that were there all the time, those that came for a visit, those that called, texted, "Facebooked" and e-mailed. Thanks to the high school girls, the Princeton girls, Ryan's rowing buddies and my Seattle friends, and especially to my co-survivors who helped guide me through and offered invaluable advice. I am so thankful you were on my team and rooting for me.

Special thanks to Dede Cummings for believing in this manuscript (perhaps more than I did at times) and guiding me on the path to publication. Your own story has inspired me and I admire how you continue to help others.

And my last shout out is to my treatment team at the Seattle Cancer Care Alliance (Dr. Calhoun, Dr. Ellis, Dr. Wang, Dr. Neligan, Dr. Lehman, Dr. DeMartini, and Dr. Hickman; along with nurses Cathy, Sandy, and Jeanne; as well as Chaplin Deborah Jarvis; the radiation technologists; residents; and medical students). You guys saved me. I'm so thankful you do your jobs so well.